D0460000

The End-of-Life
Namaste
Care Program
for People with Dementia

The End-of-Life

Namaste

Care Program
for People with Dementia

Joyce Simard, M.S.W.

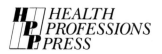
HEALTH
PROFESSIONS
PRESS

Baltimore • London • Sydney

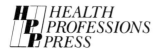

HEALTH PROFESSIONS PRESS

Health Professions Press, Inc.
Post Office Box 10624
Baltimore, Maryland 21285-0624

www.healthpropress.com

Typeset by Barton Matheson Willse & Worthington, Baltimore, Maryland.
Manufactured in the United States of America by Versa Press, East Peoria, Illinois.
Cover design by Mindy Dunn.

The information provided in this book is in no way meant to substitute for a medical practitioner's advice or expert opinion. Readers should consult a medical practitioner if they are interested in more information. This book is sold without warranties of any kind, express or implied, and the publisher and author disclaim any liability, loss, or damage caused by the contents of this book.

All of the case studies described in this book are based on the author's actual experiences, but the names and identifying details have been changed to protect privacy. Exceptions include EPOCH Senior Healthcare (pp. 8–9), the Vermont Veterans Home (Chapter 6; Appendix G), and Matthew and Celia Wilk (throughout), whose stories recounted in this book are real and whose permission for this use is gratefully acknowledged.

Library of Congress Cataloging-in-Publication Data
Simard, Joyce
    The end-of-life namaste care program for people with dementia / by Joyce Simard.
      p.   cm.
    Includes bibliographical references.
    ISBN 978-1-932529-34-0 (alk. paper)
    1. Dementia—Patients—Nursing home care.   2. Terminally ill—Nursing home care.   3. Spiritual care (Medical care) I. Title.
    [DNLM: 1. Alzheimer Disease—nursing.   2. Dementia—nursing.
    3. Holistic Health.   4. Terminal Care—methods. WY 152 S588e 2007]
RC521.S57 2007
616.8'31029—dc22
                                         2007023163

Contents

About the Author

Working from Florida and the Czech Republic, **Joyce Simard, M.S.W.**, provides consulting services to skilled nursing centers and assisted living communities worldwide. She earned her bachelor of arts in sociology/social work at Ithaca College in New York and her master's of social work at the University of Minnesota.

In addition to Namaste Care, she developed The Memory Enhancement Program (MEP), a unique program for individuals experiencing memory loss above and beyond what is normal for their age and education. Residents in nursing centers, assisted living, and independent living communities who do not need a secured Alzheimer's unit benefit from this program.

Ms. Simard is author of a children's book about aging and dementia, *The Magic Tape Recorder* (2007). She is also an internationally recognized speaker who has presented both to families of people with dementia and to health care professionals in the United States, Europe, Australia, and several cities in Asia on topics including Understanding Alzheimer's Disease, Finding Joy in the Caregiving Experience, and Staff Participation in Meaningful Activities. In addition, she provides in-service training on a variety of subjects, including hospice, bereavement, comfort care, and activity programs for people with dementia.

Ms. Simard's inspiring presentations have led her to be selected as the keynote or featured speaker at many professional conferences. She is known for bringing humor and a light touch to serious subjects, and she teaches through stories of real experiences from her more than 20 years in health care.

For more information, visit the Web site www.joycesimard.com.

Foreword

Despite significant progress being made in our understanding of the pathological processes involved in Alzheimer's disease, there is still no effective treatment that would prevent it, cure it, or stop its inevitable progression. We are therefore faced with the need to care for individuals throughout the course of this and other progressive degenerative dementias.

Many improvements have been made in the care of individuals with mild and moderate dementia. These include support groups for newly diagnosed individuals and for their caregivers, increased availability of home care, and the establishment of special care dementia units in congregate care facilities. Less attention has been paid, however, to care provided to individuals with severe dementia. Often, in fact, these individuals in the advanced stages of the disease are discharged from special care dementia units because they may not benefit from the programs that are available there. The need for programs that would be suitable for individuals with severe and terminal dementia is strong if we are to prevent them from progressing into a vegetative state and help them to continue to enjoy personal contact and stimulation.

The End-of-Life Namaste Care Program for People with Dementia describes an enlightened program that has been successfully implemented in several nursing homes and hospice organizations. Namaste Care strives to maintain the highest quality of life possible for individuals with severe and terminal dementia. This care involves the creation of a special room that provides a quiet, peaceful environment for residents in the last stage of their disease. Meaningful activities are individualized for each resident and a continuous presence of staff member(s) provides both physical and sensory stimulation. This "high-touch" care can be taught to all staff as well as family members. The family members, particularly, appreciate the attention given to their loved ones.

It is my hope that publication of this book will stimulate many more nursing homes and hospices to pay greater attention to individuals with advanced and terminal dementia. *The End-of-Life Namaste Care Program for People with Dementia* may serve as an important road map in this effort because it describes in detail how the program can be implemented, how the Namaste Care team is established, how an appropriate Namaste Care environment is created, and what the day's activities could be. In addition, the book discusses decision making at the end of life and what is meant by "comfort care." An understanding of death and dying and the need for care after death are also provided. Appendixes present templates of useful documents needed for establishing a Namaste Care program.

Namaste Care, as described in this book, provides residents and their families with quality care that addresses not only physical but also emotional and spiritual needs. It reminds us that individuals with advanced dementia should not be isolated in their rooms, but need to live their last days in a pleasant environment receiving loving care from all staff and families.

Ladislav Volicer, M.D., Ph.D., F.A.A.N., F.G.S.A.

Retired Clinical Director
Geriatric Research Education and
Clinical Center (GRECC)
Veterans Administration Hospital
Bedford, Massachusetts

Preface

"I have lost myself."

Auguste D.

On November 4, 1906, Dr. Alois Alzheimer gave a lecture in which he described Auguste D., a 51-year-old woman with symptoms of a progressive, cognitive impairment. He had been puzzled that a woman so young exhibited symptoms usually seen in those much older. After Auguste's death in April of 1906, Dr. Alzheimer had performed an autopsy on her brain to try to determine the reason for her unusual behavior. When the brain samples were placed under a microscope, he discovered the plaques and neurofibrillary tangles that are now recognized as the markers of the disease that became named after this researcher: Alzheimer's disease (AD). At the time, however, his lecture was virtually ignored by his colleagues and the material was deemed "not appropriate for a publication" (Maurer, Volk, & Gerbaldo, 1997).

A hundred years after this lecture, Dr. Alzheimer's name is famous and he is internationally recognized as the physician who discovered AD, a condition that at the beginning of the 21st century affects 5.3 million Americans and costs the U.S. health care system $100 billion per year (Alzheimer's Association, 2007). AD is the fourth leading cause of death and is the disease most greatly feared by people older than 55 (MetLife Foundation, 2006).

According to a quote taken from her medical records, Auguste D. cried out to Dr. Alzheimer, "I have lost myself." This lament is as relevant today to the millions of people struggling with AD as it was to this woman a century ago. Another entry in Auguste D.'s files quotes her husband as being upset with his wife's accusations of infidelity. Upsetting behavior such as this continues to distress present-day spouses, who are often bewildered by accusations of being unfaithful. Unfortunately, the despair and confusion surrounding AD continue.

Auguste D. was placed in a mental asylum. Today, thankfully, there are many more options for caring for individuals with AD. Services such as adult day services, home health care aides, housekeeping services, and respite care are available to offer families periods of relief from the exhausting caregiving responsibilities that accompany AD. If she lived today, perhaps Auguste D. would be able to live in an assisted living community that specializes in the care of people with early and moderate dementia. When her dementia progressed, Auguste D. would spend the last years of her life in a skilled nursing facility that offers a special care unit. Hospice might be a part of her care in the last months of her life, and bereavement services would be offered to her husband.

From diagnosis to death, both family and professional care partners now have access to a vast array of services and information on behavioral approaches and medical treatments to help make life easier for the person with AD. We know how to help the person with early and moderate dementia maintain a quality of life while living at home or in a health care setting. The Alzheimer's Association has published recommendations for assisted living residences and nursing facilities to improve the quality of dementia care (Alzheimer's Association, 2005), and some states regulate special care units, which are dementia-specific units.

The need nevertheless remains for increased focus on care for nursing facility residents with *advanced dementia*. The Alzheimer's Association has determined that end-of-life care needs more attention from researchers as well as from health care practitioners (Volicer, 2005) as they strive to improve care in residential settings. Nursing facilities tend to focus on medical care for residents with advanced dementia: monitoring vital signs and dispensing medication. Residents are well groomed, changed, and fed. But what is the quality of life?

In some nursing facilities, residents with advanced dementia are grouped around the nurses' station so that they can be observed. Other residents with advanced dementia are isolated in their rooms. Some nurses believe that the kindest way to care for residents with advanced dementia who are no longer ambulatory is to leave them in bed. They spend the rest of their lives in one room, alone for the majority of the day—their voices stilled by the disease. Because they no longer cry out "I'm here" or "Help me," they are easy to forget in the busy life of a nursing facility. In some respects, they become invisible.

These individuals deserve the right to be acknowledged and to be in the presence of others. Our ears must hear their silent cries and we must find ways to continue to acknowledge their person-hood with respect and loving care. I developed the Namaste pro-gram to bring an improved quality of life to nursing facility resi-dents in the last stage of a dementing disease. *Namaste* (pronounced *nah-ma-stā*) is a Hindu term meaning "to honor the spirit within," a perfect name for a program designed to acknowledge the person first, not the disease. The Namaste program removes the isolation surrounding these residents and invites them to a place filled with love and the presence of others.

It has been my great fortune to work with people who have helped to grow this one idea into an ever-evolving experience that has increased the quality of life of whomever it touches. As my con-cept of Namaste grew, the name changed to Namaste Care to en-compass the many additional services offered as part of the pro-gram. This book was written in the hope that you, the reader, will be inspired to enhance the care that is provided to residents with advanced dementia in your facility.

The book is personal, a documented journey of more than 25 years in long-term care. This journey reflects the various changes in how nursing facilities have cared for residents with memory loss. In this book, you will find step-by-step advice on how to start a simi-lar program in your facility. Vignettes of actual experiences appear throughout the book. As you no doubt have often seen, the humor-ous side of life in long-term care makes a sometimes difficult job less stressful. I hope that you will smile as you read about some of my less-than-stellar ideas.

As more residents live longer with AD, the number of individ-uals with advanced dementia grows. Let us join hands and hearts and give a voice to residents who can no longer speak. Let us gather these residents to be in the presence of others. Quality of life is a right for all people. Namaste Care is one way to make this a reality for residents with advanced dementia. Please join me in making the commitment to raise the standards of end-of-life care for people with advanced dementia.

Joyce Simard, M.S.W.
July 2007

Acknowledgments

The acknowledgments could easily be as long as the book. Many people, including residents, professional health care staff, and family members, have contributed to the formulation of Namaste Care over the years. A special thank you goes to Celia Wilk, wife of Matthew, who gave me permission to share how Namaste Care helped to fill Matthew's last months and days with moments of joy. His death was, in fact, the force that led me to write this book.

Without support from the past and present administrators, department managers, and the incredible staff of the Vermont Veterans Home (VVH), Namaste Care might still be an unrealized dream. The first Namaste Care program was up and running within 30 days of the administrator's approval. It happened quickly because of the commitment of many dedicated individuals at VVH. Mary Longtin, who began providing Namaste Care before it had a name, is one of those people who touches your life and leaves an indelible mark. She continues to be an inspiration to all whose lives she touches. Activity Director Michele Burgess, Dementia Program Director Christina Cosgrove, and Director of Nursing Marlene Restino put a great deal of time and effort into getting Namaste Care started. Words cannot describe the commitment of the B Wing staff. Under the leadership of charge nurse Jennie LaBrake, Namaste Care has become nationally and internationally recognized as an innovative program of care for nursing facility residents with advanced dementia.

Under the dynamic leadership of CEO Joanna Cormac-Burt, EPOCH Senior Healthcare in Waltham, Massachusetts, has made a commitment to offer Namaste Care in all of its nursing facilities with dementia units. With strong support from Regional Vice President of Operations Kim Sciacca, corporate nurses Barbara Baker and Karen Roberts, and the staff at EPOCH Senior Healthcare of Chestnut Hill, Norton, Brewster, and Harwich, Namaste Care has raised the bar for providing quality care for residents with advanced dementia in Massachusetts. Many of the excellent learning experiences in this book were made possible by the devotion of the leaders of EPOCH Senior Healthcare to provide excellent care for their residents, and by their good humor as we made Namaste Care a reality in a very short time. Thank you, all!

My gratitude to friend and colleague Sally Zinn Brunworth, a leader in the long-term care field for many years, for her help in ensuring the accuracy of the medical and nursing issues covered in the text. She took time out from her much-deserved retirement to read and give valuable feedback on the book. Kudos also to Joanne Pollack, who read every word to make sure every comma was in place and that even a layperson could easily understand the book.

Namaste Care would never have been written if it were not for the loving support of Ladislav Volicer. His cheerleading, methodical review of all chapters, and understanding of the medical issues that accompany dementia care were invaluable.

Finally, this book would never reach so many health care professionals if Mary Magnus, Director of Publications for Health Professions Press, had not taken a chance on this unknown author. Thank you, Mary.

To Ladislav Volicer, M.D., Ph.D.

A pioneer in quality-of-life issues for individuals with advanced dementia.

*His research has inspired health care professionals
throughout the world to humanize end-of-life care.*

CHAPTER 1

The Beginning

We never know how our lives will be shaped by events that initially seem insignificant but are actually profound turning points. My first interview for a social work position took place in Ithaca, New York, in 1978. Walking into a very old nursing facility, formerly a rehabilitation center for children with polio, my thoughts were something like: *This is not for me; this will have to be a temporary position.* All of the residents looked so old and disabled and sad. My focus was children, a population that had a future. But as I have learned, sometimes the hard way, life has a way of leading you in the direction of "the road less traveled."

As part of the interview, the administrator gave me a tour of the building as residents were being gathered for lunch. He asked me to help take the residents into the dining room; of course, I readily agreed. My first efforts to move a wheelchair did not work. Tugging and then trying to lift it produced no forward movement. No one told me that wheelchairs have brakes. Needless to say, this new social worker had a lot to learn!

In spite of my ineptness, I was hired and began a career that would turn out to be my life's work, my mission, and my joy. The main responsibility in this position was admissions, keeping the beds full. Then, because of my eagerness to get to know residents and the lack of time in which to do it, I began to lead the group sessions with residents' families, trying to understand what they were feeling as their loved ones were admitted to a nursing facility. The facility must have had residents with dementia, but looking back, I do not remember working with them.

It was not until 1979, when our family was transferred to Minnesota, that my interest in residents with dementia surfaced. At Westwood Nursing Home in Saint Louis Park, Minnesota, I assumed responsibility for the "dreaded" second floor, where most of the residents had what we now know as Alzheimer's disease (AD) or a related dementia. Residents were diagnosed with senile dementia, pre-senile dementia, or organic brain syndrome. Sometimes the medical records completely ignored the memory loss and just addressed the person's medical problems. These residents were hidden from the tours we gave to families because we did not want anyone to be frightened by the behavior sometimes exhibited on this floor. We also saw this exile as a way to protect these residents from escaping.

Social workers did not enjoy working on the second floor because they could not use the skills they had learned. Staff members were puzzled when the residents would not listen or follow directions. Residents would repeatedly wander or disrobe in public. We diagnosed them as having problem behaviors and recommended medicating them. Sometimes, we sent them to a psychiatric unit of the local hospital. Counseling was impossible because of the residents' severe memory loss. Nonetheless, this floor became my responsibility. With little understanding of why a resident could not remember that her mother had died years ago or that she did not have to go home to care for her "children" who were now 40 years old, I was mystified about how to provide social work services to my clientele.

We provided what we thought was good care. Residents with dementia were clean, well fed, and attended to medically. A few activity programs offered diversion in bits and pieces, but activity staff struggled to find ways to entertain residents with memory loss. Because they might "act out" during programs, they received fewer hours of dedicated activity services than other residents. The "oriented" residents, who appreciated being involved in activities and were very vocal, were simply more rewarding to work with. Clearly, we struggled with what to do with a group of residents who lived in another reality.

At this time, many residents in nursing facilities looked more like today's assisted living residents. They were interested in crafts and current events and loved spending time with staff. It was not unusual to have residents who just wanted to talk waiting for me when I came in each morning.

All levels of staff were taught to use reality orientation (RO) at all times. This approach taught that it was important to constantly remind residents of their surroundings, the time, the place, the person, the *truth*! We believed that saying the same thing over and over would help residents with memory loss live in the present. When a resident asked where he was or said that she wanted to go home, we replied, "You are in a nursing home, your children are grown, and you do not need to fix dinner for them. Your children are adults with their own homes." Many residents looked for their mothers. We would tell them the devastating news that their mother had died 20 years ago. This perpetually "new" information was shocking and upsetting to them. Here is a recollection of one of my first encounters with a resident who must have had AD:

SALLY

While getting to know residents on the second floor, a woman in her eighties approached me and asked if I had seen her mother. My tender and compassionate response was that her mother had passed away. She, of course, was shocked at this information and dissolved into tears. Within 5 minutes, she approached me again with the same question; my response was the same, her mother had died. Once again, she cried over the "recent" loss of her mother. This was quite demoralizing. After all, my job was to help the residents feel good, not cause them to cry. When Sally approached me the third time with the same question, my gut reaction was to try a different response. Not quite knowing what this line of questioning would produce, I asked her to describe her mother. With a big smile, she told me what her mother looked like and what a wonderful mother she was. We proceeded to have a delightful conversation about all kinds of things, and when our visit was over, I reassured her that I would look for her mother. The resident walked away very happy that someone would help her. Somehow my question, which had no basis in reality, reached this woman. At least for a moment, she was at peace.

I decided that the best approach to working with residents on this floor was not to use RO. They needed a new approach to help them live in their world.

CHANGES IN DEMENTIA CARE

Nursing facilities providing care for the growing population of residents with dementia began to change in the 1980s as new approaches began to emerge. Nursing facility owners also realized that dementia care was a good business. Special care units (SCUs) emerged; these were secured areas within a facility that provided special activities for residents with dementia and special educational programs for staff. It was an exciting time as the long-term care industry explored ways to help residents with dementia maintain quality in their lives.

During this time, a social worker named Naomi Feil (1982) introduced Validation Therapy. After attending one of her workshops, my excitement could hardly be contained. Someone was finally giving advice on working with residents with memory loss and an altered sense of reality. Why not join their journey rather than try to drag them into our world? Validation Therapy offered staff members an approach to help residents with memory loss live happier lives. Blanch is just one example of a resident who benefited from the shift from RO to Validation Therapy.

BLANCH

Blanch, a widow in her seventies with two grown sons and grandchildren, believed that she was on vacation. Every morning she thanked the staff for the wonderful hospitality but said her husband was picking her up so she could go home to care for her two small children. The staff hugged her, told her how they had enjoyed having her visit, and then suggested that she have breakfast while waiting for her husband to arrive. Blanch happily walked to the dining room and forgot about going home. The next day it would all start again.

Years ago, Blanch would have been distressed day after day as she was told the "truth": that her husband was deceased, her sons were grown, and she was living in a nursing facility. Using Validation Therapy supported Blanch's belief that she was on vacation with her friends; what a pleasant way for Blanch to spend her days!

In time, the Alzheimer's Association was formed. Founded in 1980, it emerged as the leading force in awakening the public's awareness of AD. Beginning with a few family members and health care professionals, the Association grew to become a respected organization with 82 chapters nationwide. The Alzheimer's Association is dedicated to enhancing the quality of life of all people affected by AD and related disorders through advocacy, education, and support systems, while also promoting research efforts (Alzheimer's Association, 2007).

As the number of people with AD grew, so did the scope of services and programs offered by the Alzheimer's Association. Health care professionals were beginning to realize that the number of residents in nursing facilities who had memory loss was significant and growing, and that they needed more information on how to treat and care for this special population. Articles on AD started to appear in journals, and research studies were initiated on a variety of care issues related to residents with AD and the burdens felt by their families.

In 1990, my career took another turn when the Hillhaven Corporation, a leader in the care of residents with Alzheimer's disease, hired me. Under the leadership of Nancy Orr-Rainey, a department was created to develop SCUs (Orr-Rainey, 1994). These units were secured so residents would be in a safe, controlled environment. SCUs were designed with country kitchens so the ladies could feel at home, help prepare a meal, or sit at the kitchen table. Office spaces were established for men who had "work" to do. Outside courtyards were built so residents could enjoy being outside, planting gardens, or watching birds as they flocked around the bird feeders. Living rooms were arranged so that games could be played and families could visit in comfortable surroundings.

Nursing facilities realized that special dementia units were good for their business. They recognized that SCUs with quality programming had a healthy census with a waiting list. When the emergence of assisted living residences began to erode their private-pay census, many nursing facility companies found that a specialized dementia unit had the greatest potential to attract new private-pay residents. Most nursing facility companies lose money on Medicaid residents; their ability to attract private-pay residents helps keep the companies solvent.

Several years ago, the large nursing facility company that employed me as its National Director of Alzheimer's Services held a "nursing facility of the future" meeting. When asked my thoughts on what the building should look like, I described creating a small, secured wing for the few oriented residents and devoting the rest of the building to people with various stages of memory loss. Staff members in nursing facilities today say that at least 80% of those residents who are not on the rehabilitation unit have some significant memory loss. In the relatively new assisted living industry, more than 68% of residents have a diagnosis of dementia (Maust et al., 2006). Many assisted living companies now build some communities that exclusively cater to residents with dementia.

My first experience in assisted living was with Marriott Senior Living Services, where I was fortunate to be able to help design all aspects of their SCUs. It was a pleasure to work with interior designers who were responsive to the needs of residents with dementia and created homelike surroundings that help residents know what to do in a variety of spaces. We noticed that when the environment looked like a large home or a hotel, residents were less anxious and seemed more at home. They could identify the living room with its couches and television set, felt comfortable relaxing with other residents in the country kitchen, and clearly knew that the dining room was the place in which to eat. Marriott designed the dining rooms to look like restaurants. As a result, residents were on their best behavior, as they thought they were going out to eat. Many insisted on paying for the meal, so we developed a way for them to pay and leave a tip.

As more and more SCUs were developed, the need for a special activity program emerged. These residents needed something to do with their time. Most health care professionals agree that residents with moderate to advanced dementia rarely self-initiate meaningful activities and need continuous activity programming (Volicer et al., 2006). When a resident with dementia has nothing to do, he or she tends to engage in what are often called "problem behaviors," such as wandering into other resident's rooms, going through others' belongings and taking items, or otherwise annoying other residents and their families.

JOE

> The staff at one facility was having a very difficult time with families because of lost dentures. The nursing staff was mystified that so many dentures seemed to disappear. The solution to the problem was found when Joe died. Staff cleaning out his closet found 15 pairs of dentures that Joe had thought were his!

I have found that residents like activities that remind them of earlier times in their lives. In fact, finding ways to keep residents involved in the "life" of the unit became my specialty. I found that some women like folding laundry or washing dishes. Mothers like rocking babies and folding diapers. Men like having office work to do.

As nursing facilities grew more aware of the specialized needs of the residents with dementia, educational programs were offered to help staff understand how to provide care for residents with memory loss. Many training films and educational materials became available for health care professionals and family care partners. The Alzheimer's Association has taken the lead in developing educational programs for professionals and families. Today, basic Alzheimer's education is part of the orientation program in many skilled nursing facilities and assisted living communities. Many states now mandate training in AD for all staff.

NEW APPROACHES TO PROVIDING DEMENTIA CARE

With her Validation approach, Naomi Feil (2002) opened the door to a new way of caring for people with memory loss. Others have followed with a variety of approaches that continue to improve quality of life for people with dementia. Virginia Bell and David Troxel (1996, 2003) wrote about becoming a *best friend* to someone with AD. Tom Kitwood's (1998) *person-centered therapy* recognizes the importance of the individual first, the disease second. Cameron Camp developed Montessori-based activities as a rehabilitation approach to the treatment of dementia (Orsulic-Jeras, Judge, & Camp, 2000). In 1994, Bill Thomas publicly declared what we all knew, that nursing facilities were filled with residents who felt lonely, helpless, and bored; this statement has helped to humanize nursing facilities (Thomas, 2004). Betsy Brawley (1997), an interior designer whose mother had AD, wrote about creating dementia environments that support life. All of these innovators have increased health care professionals' knowledge about how to help people with AD live with their disease.

The Pioneer Network gave birth to the notion of *culture change* that is sweeping the country. This movement began in 1997 when a group of "pioneering" resident advocates and health care professionals agreed it was time to join forces to transform nursing facilities into places offering person-directed care that restored control to elders and their caregivers (Pioneer Network, 2006). The concept of culture change has come to mean a transformational change in a facility's values, practices, and day-to-day care culture. It has translated into changes in many of the nursing facilities in which I work, with positive results for both residents and staff. The following examples of culture change have helped remind the facility's staff members why they chose to work in a nursing facility.

EPOCH SENIOR HEALTHCARE

To get department managers out of their offices and away from their paperwork, EPOCH Senior Healthcare of Harwich, Massachusetts, decided that everyone had to lead at least one resident activity each month. Now, the Director of Nursing plays the piano and leads a sing-a-long. The administrator meets with residents to discuss her favorite subject, cooking; her group chooses a recipe from her cookbooks and then prepares the dish. The maintenance director leads a men's group called Guess What This Is?; he shows a tool and has the men guess how it is used. Both staff and residents have come to feel they know each other better by getting together outside of their usual roles and in a more casual setting.

Another EPOCH Senior Healthcare facility in Brewster, Massachusetts, is transforming one of its traditional, 30-year-old units into a *neighborhood* by hiding the nursing station, making the bathroom look more homelike with colorful shower curtains and pictures of old-fashioned bathtubs, and transforming the day room into a country kitchen.

Another example of the changes occurring in nursing facilities is the Nursing Home Quality Initiative of the Centers for Medicare and Medicaid Services (CMS). This initiative promotes the transformation of nursing facilities from institutional to person-centered care models (CMS, 2002). I also hear reports that surveyors are no longer satisfied with seeing a room full of residents in an activity. Now they want to know if residents had a choice in attending the program and whether they are engaged in the activity. A simple head count is not enough, especially if many participants are sleeping.

When Namaste Care was first introduced in Vermont, surveyors started suggesting that other nursing facilities send staff to observe the program. The surveyors were amazed and wanted others to see that meaningful activities could be provided for residents with advanced dementia.

With no cure in sight and the average life expectancy increasing (age is the greatest risk factor for AD), greater awareness of the need for specialized Alzheimer's services has emerged. Adult day service centers have become an option for families who choose to provide care at home and need respite during the day. Along with this service, home health companies are providing specialized services to families of clients with dementia as they meet the challenges of keeping their loved ones at home. The care of people with AD is a thriving business and we have begun the exciting process that will ultimately make nursing facilities places in which individuals, regardless of their physical or cognitive status, can live surrounded by caring staff.

PEOPLE WITH ALZHEIMER'S DISEASE FIND THEIR VOICES

Since 1994, when Ronald Reagan wrote his poignant letter telling the American people that he had Alzheimer's disease, it seems to be easier for people with AD and their families to talk about the experience of living with the disease. Families are writing books on various aspects of caring for someone with dementia. Newly diagnosed individuals are coming forward to speak about the disease; many are outspoken advocates for more research funds and quality care. Richard Taylor (2007), a former psychologist who was diagnosed with early AD, is a crusader for the newly diagnosed person with AD. He established a large electronic network and e-mailed the following message on January 24, 2007: "Stand up! So as not to become a victim of your own silence. Speak for yourself and those who will follow. Ask Carers and Friends to do the same. Today will never be here again. Time is of the Essence! Use it wisely!!! Tell as many people as possible your perceptions of your interactions with professionals, with carers, with friends, with strangers, with your government. They won't change unless they know, and they can't know unless and until you SPEAK UP! Seek to create a Palpable Sense of Change and of urgency! Join a Crusade, Now! Be a Crusader, Now! Lead a Crusade, Now!" He is one of many people with early diagnosed AD who are raising their voices to be heard at professional gatherings and in the halls of Congress. They are demanding that money be spent to find a cure. People with AD from around the world have joined together with a common cause: to live in a world without AD.

Millions of dollars are spent each year on research to find the cause and risk factors for AD. The cures, however, continue to be elusive. Medications are now available to slow the progression of the disease and new ones continue to appear fairly regularly. Every year, we inch closer to finding the reasons why some people develop Alzheimer's disease and why others do not. When we know why, perhaps we can short-circuit the process and eliminate this disease. Until that day arrives, the number of people with dementia grows at an alarming rate; almost 50% of those older than 85 years of age develop AD (Evans et al., 1989). If we do not find a way to prevent or cure AD, it may bankrupt our health care system.

Prevention has become the new battle cry of the Alzheimer's Association. In response to the aging baby boomers' fear of developing AD, the Association launched a campaign, "Maintain Your Brain," with the message to "Use your brain, exercise, and live a healthy lifestyle" (Alzheimer's Association, 2006). How lovely it would be if my great grandchildren could live without the fear of developing AD. My dream is that one day hardly anyone will remember what AD even was. Those of us who care for people with AD would be gloriously out of work!

CREATING NAMASTE CARE

Namaste Care was created in the spring of 2003, but the seeds had been planted years before. In 1981, while getting my master's degree in social work at the University of Minnesota and working part time in Westwood Nursing Home, my path crossed with a very important person. Robert Fulton, Ph.D., was a sociology professor who had studied in London with Dame Cicely Sanders, who began the modern hospice movement. He offered a course on the hospice movement that introduced me to this special way of caring for people who are dying.

My first thoughts were that hospice was a great concept for residents in nursing facilities who were dying alone and in pain. How to manage pain was not as well understood as it is today. Pain medication was not administered until the resident complained. Then it took some time to take effect and was not administrated again until the pain reappeared. This vicious cycle of pain kept many residents uncomfortable for many hours of the day and night.

In addition, the qualifications for the Medicare hospice benefit required the patient to have a "home" and "family caregiver." A nursing facility did not qualify on either count. Believing that *there is more than one way to skin a cat* (or get around a regulation), I worked with the nursing facility staff to develop a hospice-like approach ourselves.

With Professor Fulton's support and with guidance from the local hospice center, we began our own end-of-life care. This would not have happened without the dynamic leadership of administrator Cheryl Nybo, fellow social worker Michael McDonough, and the great staff at Westwood Nursing Home. This incredible team believed that people should not die alone and in pain, so we changed the way our residents spent their last days. Hospice nurses helped with pain management according to what we knew about decreasing pain at that time, and we recruited alert, oriented residents to sit by the bedsides of dying residents, giving them comfort.

Sitting by the bedside of the dying was a time-honored tradition for the older generation and was not feared by them. One resident told me that in doing this service she finally felt worthwhile—that she still could do something that mattered. I'll never forget the look on one resident's face as she struggled into the room to take her turn at the bedside. She was as big as a minute and very frail. At my suggestion that maybe this was too much for her, she pulled herself up to her full four-foot-two height and declared that she was perfectly capable and to mind my own business! I quickly backed out of the room.

It was not just other residents who sat with the dying. We enlisted everyone's help. Staff members were encouraged to do their paperwork and charting by the bedside of dying residents, just to be present for them. The dietary department made popsicles and lollipops for the residents to suck to help prevent the dry mouth that can be a problem at the end of life. The maintenance man took his truck to a resident's house, packed up her china cabinet with figurines she had collected all her life, and reassembled it in her room so that her last days could be spent looking at her treasures. One resident wanted to attend religious services but was in too much pain to leave her bed, so staff members pushed her, bed and all, to the service!

Before this time, hospice care was viewed as appropriate only for residents who were verbal and could express feelings about dying. The residents with dementia were not even considered appropriate for this program. That belief has changed. We now know that conversation at the end of life is not necessary and may not be desired; many residents just want to know that someone is there and that they are not alone.

Years passed, and finally Medicare recognized nursing facility residents as eligible for the Medicare hospice benefit (Appendix A). Few residents, however, elected to use the benefit, usually just those who had cancer and were alert and oriented. Hospice workers were familiar with these patients; they knew how to care for them physically and emotionally, but hospice workers were still not comfortable caring for residents with dementia. My attempts to get my employers interested in hospice care were never very successful.

In 1994, my path crossed with Ladislav Volicer, M.D., Ph.D., the Clinical Director of the Geriatric Research, Education and Clinical Center at the Edith Nourse Rogers Memorial Veterans Hospital in Bedford, Massachusetts. Dr. Volicer was the Medical Director of the Dementia Special Care Unit and pioneered the hospice approach to care for patients with late-stage dementia. His research has systematically evaluated the effects of implementation of palliative care options and has led to the development of policies to guide hospice care that have affected U.S. public policy and the Medicare hospice benefit for individuals with advanced dementia. Dr. Volicer is a recognized expert in many medical aspects of palliative care and a strong supporter of Namaste Care.

Using the work of Dr. Volicer and his colleagues, we developed the Bethany Program for Hillhaven. Under the guidance of Nancy Orr-Rainey, we tried with limited success to interest the nursing facility and local hospice center in forming partnerships. We included residents with dementia in the mix of those we believed would qualify for the Medicare hospice benefit. Unfortunately, it continues to be a struggle to get anyone with dementia accepted into hospice care. Even today, only 7.5% of residents who access the benefit have a diagnosis of AD (National Center for Health Statistics, 2006). The requirement for doctors to make a prognosis of "6 months to live" seems to inhibit referrals of dementia patients to hospice. Many physicians are not as enlightened as Dr. Volicer; they believe that hospice care for someone with dementia is a waste of taxpayers' dollars.

In 2001, I began to consult with a nursing facility in Bennington, Vermont. My role as a consultant was to develop a unique program for residents on the secured dementia unit. The first program we developed was "The Club," a program of continuous activities that proved that helping residents to engage in meaningful activities throughout their waking hours produces positive results (Simard & Volicer, 2002). The Club helped decrease falls, the use of psychotropic medication, and social isolation. Residents gained weight, and staff and family satisfaction significantly increased. The Club also helped to fill empty beds. The unit filled quickly and began to boast a waiting list. However, even when residents were so advanced in their disease that they did not seem to benefit from the continuous programming, families did not want them to leave the unit. C Wing had become special not only because of its excellent care but also because of The Club. We needed to create another special program that would offer a different type of programming for residents who no longer could benefit from The Club and entice families to move their loved ones off C Wing when the time came. The fact is, in many SCUs, when a resident enters the advanced stage of Alzheimer's disease, he or she is moved off the unit to another area of the facility. Most assisted living communities must move residents with advanced dementia out of their building when the resident is no longer able to ambulate and needs total care; assisted living is not usually staffed to provide the level of care needed by residents with advanced dementia, even when hospice is involved.

The administrator at the Bennington facility asked me to create a unique program for residents with advanced dementia. His vision was to expand the dementia program without simply recreating another club. A wing on one side of the nurse's station became the location for a new program, "Namaste." The programming that was developed was based on some of the creative techniques that Mary Longtin, a restorative aide, had been using on C Wing with residents with advanced dementia. With support of the administrator, all levels of staff, Director of Nursing Marlene Restino, Charge Nurse Jennie LaBrake, Dementia Program Director Christina Cosgrove, Activity Director Michele Burgess, and the staff of C Wing, we began creating the Namaste program.

With no budget, only an admonition to keep the costs as low as possible, we started Namaste in an activity room made to look less institutional with Goodwill furniture and donations of plants, quilts, and other old but interesting items. Using the amazing insight and talents of Mary Longtin, the first dedicated Namaste Care specialist, programming started with the basics of good nursing care. The residents' expressions told us that they enjoyed hand and foot massages. Other pleasurable activities included listening to music, inhaling the scent of lavender, and receiving gentle touches. The presence of others, especially the soft murmuring of voices, seemed to lower residents' anxiety. We realized that we could make a positive difference in the lives of residents who had shown little response to activities in The Club. Their families noticed a positive change in their loved ones and were delighted with the attention given to this new program. They told us that visiting time was easier when they sat in the Namaste room. Team members on the Namaste unit were proud of this new approach. Everyone appeared so satisfied, and it was so simple: A caring touch and being with others created a calming atmosphere for the dying residents. It seems that we have a great deal to learn about living from our care of the dying.

Teach Me to Die

Teach me to die
Hold on to my hand
I have so many questions
Things I don't understand
Teach me to die
Give me all you can give
If you'll teach me of dying
I will teach you to live

Deanna Edwards

Staff and family who were involved with this first Namaste program were so pleased that we realized it needed to be spread beyond the confines of this one facility. Christina, Michele, Dr. Volicer, and I began speaking about the program at conferences. Dr. Volicer and I presented the Namaste program on speaking engagements in Australia and Asia. People would often remark that no one else was offering this specialized care and would ask where they could find more information about it. I was not comfortable with the idea of writing a book, but then my presence at the death of Matthew Wilk changed everything.

Matthew's Story

Matthew was part of Namaste for several months before he died. I had seen the pleasure on his face when he was placed in a comfortable lounge chair and offered orange slices and lollipops. He was in the presence of other residents who were also in the last stages of dementia-related illnesses, not isolated in his room or asleep in The Club program. He spent the majority of the day with caring Namaste team members, in a room filled with beautiful music and the scent of lavender drifting through the air. Namaste team members offered Matthew a variety of meaningful activities, such as receiving hand and foot massages, listening to the sounds of nature, and hearing gentle conversations. Matthew spent the last months of his life in this comforting place with his wife, Celia, often at his side.

Matthew Wilk died on July 12, 2004. Matthew was a husband to Celia for 56 years, a father of five, a retired transformer specialist for General Electric for 35 years, and a person who had lived with dementia for 6 years.

Because of his participation in the Namaste Care program, Matthew's last weeks could have been sad; they were not. Matthew's last days could have been heartbreaking; they were not. Matthew's last hours could have been distressing; they were not. Matthew's death could have been devastating; it was not. Matthew left this world with dignity, love, and compassionate care and on the wings of laughter (Simard, 2005).

Several months after Matthew's death, his wife Celia and I were sitting in the private room reserved for Namaste residents. This was the room where Matthew spent his last days, where he died. She looked around the room and gave a rueful smile at this bittersweet space, still trying to make sense of the incredible events that had taken place in this room. We realized that the passing of Matthew had made a difference in both of our lives. For Celia, it was the end of a journey for her husband who had struggled with dementia for so many years. For me, it was being present during his death and seeing how the Namaste program had taken on a life of its own and blossomed in ways I never anticipated. Namaste could really make a difference in the way people with advanced dementia lived their last days and how they died. I needed to tell its story. Just as storytellers have taught lessons of life for thousands of years, Namaste Care will be illustrated through the story of Matthew Wilk—one of his final gifts.

CHAPTER 2

What Is Namaste Care?

The word *namaste*, pronounced "nah-ma-stā," is a Hindu greeting often used in the United States by yoga instructors as a farewell to students at the end of class. Two hands are pressed together and held near the heart with the head gently bowed as the person says, "Namaste. Go in peace." The word *namaste* expresses a wish to "honor the spirit within" and was selected as the name to describe a special way of caring for nursing facility residents with advanced dementia. As the Namaste program evolved, "Care" was added to the name to describe the many ways that Namaste team members provide services and programming to residents and their families. Thus, the name of the program has officially become Namaste Care.

Namaste Care is designed to honor the spirit of nursing facility residents who have reached the stage of their disease in which they are no longer able to speak, walk, think, and reason. Namaste Care philosophy supports the belief that the spirit of residents with advanced dementia continues to live. We see the spirit in residents' eyes, their smiles, and their response to a loving touch. This is the spirit that is undaunted by disease, the spirit beyond the disease. It is the essence of a person.

Namaste

I honor the place in you
in which the entire Universe dwells,
I honor the place in you
which is of Love, of Truth, of Light and of Peace.
When you are in that place in you,
and I am in that place in me,
we are One.

Namaste Care supports the belief that each resident is unique, like a finely woven tapestry. During each stage of the disease, more threads of the tapestry are unraveled, and the fabric of each individual's life fades. When residents with advanced dementia reach a state in which they can no longer relate their life history, their personhood is compromised.

Namaste carers take pride in knowing each resident in their care and individualizing their care to each person. Namaste carers review the resident's social history; they speak to the resident's family members and friends to learn the resident's likes and dislikes. Namaste carers also share information with each other about the residents. Thus, Namaste Care team members feel a strong bond with residents in their care. Residents are respected as individuals. Care approaches are tailored to make interaction between Namaste carers and residents personal.

The staff members who provide care are given a unique title, Namaste carer, which recognizes and respects their unique knowledge and training. With the expectation that what we learn from Namaste Care will be reflected in the care received by all people with Alzheimer's disease (AD), the term *care partner* is used in place of *nursing assistant* for the remainder of this book. It equalizes the relationship between two parties and reminds all staff members, Namaste carers included, that they should always treat residents as individuals who, whenever possible, deserve to be offered choices and to be involved in their own care.

Namaste Care began as a day program of sensory activities. Residents were transported to the Namaste Care room for the entire day or part of the day. While in the room, residents were offered a variety of sensory activities by Namaste carers. Later, the program was expanded to include food and beverages; residents with advanced dementia are at risk of weight loss and dehydration and seem to enjoy taking nourishment in the Namaste Care room. Families began to enjoy visiting in the Namaste Care room as team members would give ideas on how to make their visit more enjoyable. At this stage of their disease, many residents do not recognize their loved ones. Family members say that their visits are more enjoyable when they can do something for their loved one, so they are offered ideas on how to make their visits special. For example, some family members like to feed their loved ones ice cream, others are given lotion to massage into their loved ones' hands.

Eventually, the original Namaste Care program expanded to an entire wing with a private room for the actively dying resident and his or her family. After-death care became a part of the services offered, and Namaste Care kept "blossoming."

When hospice members saw Namaste Care in action, they expressed a desire to bring their patients to the Namaste Care room and learn ways to provide meaningful activities for residents with advanced dementia. Pleas from other units in the nursing facility to include their residents in Namaste Care gave the impetus to put together a movable Namaste Care cart, which became fondly known as Namaste a la Carte.

It became apparent that Namaste Care could be provided in many settings, including assisted living communities, hospice houses, and family homes. Namaste Care can be provided by anyone who understands its philosophy and the comfort care approaches used. Most Namaste carers who have worked with the program find that activity ideas just flow when they focus on using sensory-based techniques. Anyone who can express love, offer a gentle touch, and be present for people who are embarking on the final stage of life can be a Namaste carer.

This book focuses on implementing Namaste Care in nursing facilities because this is the final home for many people with advanced dementia. As AD progresses, it becomes more and more difficult for family members to provide care in the home; likewise, assisted living communities are often not able to provide the level of care needed.

Nursing facilities are equipped for and Namaste carers are trained in providing good physical care. Facilities are challenged, however, when asked to provide meaningful activities to residents with advanced dementia. Namaste Care blends nursing care and meaningful activities to provide a holistic program that touches all aspects of a resident's life. Once the philosophy of Namaste Care is understood, the foundation is in place to operationalize Namaste Care.

THE PHILOSOPHY AND MISSION STATEMENT

The foundation of any program is an idea, a philosophy. That philosophy must be written in order to stay focused. A philosophy statement outlines beliefs and values. To help people understand the philosophy of hospice, the philosophy statement for Namaste Care was created:

Namaste Care Philosophy Statement

We believe that the spirit in each person lives regardless
of their physical and cognitive status. It is our honor
to nurture each individual through loving touch,
meaningful activities, and the presence of others. We
will do everything in our power to make the passing
on as gentle and peaceful as possible.

While the philosophy is what you believe, the mission statement is what you do.

Namaste Care Mission Statement

Namaste Care is provided by an interdisciplinary team
of compassionate and knowledgeable health care
professionals as well as families and friends. A holistic
approach to care assures that the burdens and benefits
of each medical intervention or nursing treatment are
weighed so that they support quality of life. Comfort

and pleasure are goals of Namaste Care. Every effort is
made so that the dying process is a pain-free, easy
passing surrounded by people who care.

Each nursing facility offering Namaste Care should create a unique
mission statement. A good way to have all Namaste Care team
members "buy in" to a new program is to involve them in writing
the mission statement. A facilitator should assist the team members
in fashioning their own declaration for the unit or the program.
Brief meetings should be scheduled with each shift, including staff
from all departments usually assigned to the unit or program. This
includes nursing, housekeeping, maintenance, dietary, activities,
and any auxiliary staff. All team members should be asked to state,
in their own words, their goals for the program. How should residents, their families, and staff feel when they become part of the
unit or program? The facilitator should write down any phrases,
words, and thoughts that are offered. After the meetings are completed, a draft of a mission statement is written with the help of key
managers and team members.

Consider asking the unit or program director, charge nurse,
and lead care partner to help with this project. Using the words
given by the Namaste Care team members at the meetings shows
that their ideas have been heard and that their input is valuable. The
draft mission statement should then be passed out to all team members to solicit any necessary changes or additions. When the mission statement has been approved by the majority of the team, it is
presented to the administrator. The final mission statement is
printed on high-quality paper and framed with a wide mat. Ask each
person working on the unit or program to sign the mat. The framed
mission statement is hung on the wall, a reminder to everyone that
they are entering a special place. The mission statement is also used
to orient all new team members.

OVERVIEW OF NAMASTE CARE PROGRAMMING

Namaste Care programming is a 7-day-per-week sensory-based
program that integrates nursing care and meaningful activities. The
program is situated in a designated Namaste Care room. A quiet,

welcoming aura is created in the room by lowering the lights, eliminating extraneous noise such as overhead paging, and playing soothing music. Residents are greeted by Namaste carers and placed in comfortable lounge chairs if their wheelchairs cannot be adjusted for maximum relaxation. Quilts are tucked around residents to keep them warm and secure. The Namaste carer, usually a care partner who has received special education regarding the care of residents with advanced dementia, provides a variety of meaningful activities.

Activities may include washing of feet and hands, giving massages, moisturizing the face, and gently brushing hair or moving to music. Nourishments offered include lollipops, fresh orange slices, ice cream, puddings, and nourishing shakes. Activity staff may provide reassuring sensory objects such as realistic-looking birds that chirp, wind chimes, and singing bowls. Namaste carers also provide natural items to smell, such as freshly cut grass or lilacs and objects that bring smiles to the faces of residents, such as puppets.

Residents may attend Namaste Care for the entire day or part of the day depending on their physical status. Family members and friends are encouraged to visit the Namaste Care room and often enjoy providing hand massages or holding hands with their loved ones. Alternatively, Namaste Care may be offered at the bedside with sensory items located on a cart or by hospice staff. A detailed description of the Namaste Care day can be found in Chapter 5.

COMPONENTS OF NAMASTE CARE

The Namaste Care components give it credibility and structure. They are as follows:

- Personalized mission statement
- Criteria to determine which residents would benefit from Namaste Care
- Staff selected based on the desire to work with Namaste Care
- Special education for Namaste Care team members
- Soothing and comfortable environments
- Comfort care approaches

- Programming 7 days per week in the Namaste Care room
- Grief comfort and bereavement service referrals
- Special services for the actively dying resident
- After-death care
- After-death evaluation

CRITERIA FOR RECEIVING NAMASTE CARE

In order to determine who will be served by Namaste Care, admission or participation guidelines need to be developed and written. The guidelines help staff, families, other professionals, and state surveyors understand the physical and cognitive status of the population to be served. Most of the residents in Namaste Care will have a diagnosis of an advanced irreversible dementia or similar symptoms, as well as the following:

- Inability to actively participate in activity programs
- Mini-Mental State Exam score from 0 to 7
- Difficulty communicating
- Need for assistance with most personal care
- Nonambulatory

Alzheimer's Disease

People with Alzheimer's disease (AD) are the primary participants in Namaste Care programs. AD is a progressive, irreversible brain disorder that gradually destroys a person's memory and ability to learn, reason, make judgments, communicate, and carry out daily activities. People with AD may also experience changes in their personalities and may have hallucinations and/or delusions. At this time no cure for AD is available.

It is believed that AD is caused by a number of factors, including genetic predisposition. Some families have a history of early-onset AD, and other people have genes known to increase the risk of developing AD. It is well known that age is the greatest risk factor for developing AD; the probability of having AD is almost 50% by age 85 (Alzheimer's Association, 2007).

Environmental factors such as stress, head injury, and low education are also high on the list of risk factors for developing AD (Alzheimer's Association, 2007). Research indicates that if a person is intellectually stimulated, exercises regularly, controls his or her blood pressure, and maintains low cholesterol levels, he or she lowers the chances of developing AD (Alzheimer's Association, 2007).

The first signs of AD are usually significant short-term memory loss, increased confusion, and difficulty with shopping and household tasks. A visit to a physician is necessary to rule out any reversible causes for these symptoms. As part of the diagnostic work-up, physicians will take a physical history, give the person a thorough medical exam, run laboratory tests, and conduct various neurological and memory tests. Ultimately, a diagnosis of AD is not certain until death, when an autopsy can confirm the presence of amyloid plaques and neurofibrillary tangles in the brain.

The diagnosis of AD may be complicated because of the presence of other related dementias, including vascular dementia, frontotemporal dementia, dementia with Lewy bodies, and Parkinson's disease. Although early-stage symptoms of these other dementias differ, by the advanced stage symptoms become very similar.

When a person is diagnosed with probable or possible AD, one of the several medications that show promise in slowing the progression of AD may be prescribed. The usual life span of a person with AD is 8 years, although some individuals live as long as 20 years with the disease.

Namaste Care has been designed for residents in the advanced stage of AD or a related dementia. Residents in the advanced stage of their disease are usually unable to take part in typical daily activities and will benefit from the special programming provided as part of Namaste Care.

Other Diagnoses or Conditions Suitable for Namaste Care

If the resident does not fit the criteria established for Namaste Care but nursing and activity staff struggle with providing care and meaningful activities to the resident, the most important question is,

"Will Namaste Care improve this resident's quality of life?" As the original Namaste Care program progressed, team members often suggested including residents who initially did not seem to meet the criteria for Namaste Care. Consider the story of Martha, a resident whose life was profoundly changed by Namaste Care.

MARTHA

Martha, a resident in a nursing facility, had a diagnosis of mental illness. She had been a resident for 6 years and was quite alone. Never having been married, her closest relative was a nephew who visited infrequently. Martha was one of those residents who sits in front of the nurse's station and screams "Help me!" Every facility has residents like Martha, and the staff is challenged and frustrated by them. No matter what is tried to help soothe and calm, nothing seems to work. Martha cried out for help and complained of a headache. No amount of medication seemed to help her. No amount of handholding seemed to help her. She had every imaginable test over the years, and no clinical reason for her expression of pain could be found. Very few of the nursing and activity staff were able to connect with her in a meaningful way. She was sometimes comforted by placing a cool washcloth over her forehead; when care partners had the time, they would sit by her side. Martha did not like to be touched, so giving personal care was a challenge. In desperation, staff brought her to the Namaste Care room. She was lifted from her wheelchair and placed in a comfortable lounge chair. A comforter was tucked under her chin. Then the miracle began.

Martha stopped screaming. The headache complaints ceased. She looked around the room and seemed pleased by what she saw. She still did not like to be touched by most Namaste Care team members, but she developed a very special relationship with a male care partner whom she allowed to care for her. When Martha hugged him, a beautiful expression appeared on her face; it was as if she finally had a son. Martha enjoyed sucking on lollipops and watching nature videos from her favorite chair. She seemed to appreciate the quiet environment of the Namaste Care room, and although she did not actively engage in activities, she showed that she was aware of her surroundings. The "new Martha" was easier for staff to approach. On the day she died a year later, a Namaste carer came in on her day off to hold Martha's hand. Clearly, Martha's happiest days of the last year of her life were spent in Namaste Care.

As with Martha, who didn't fit the usual profile for Namaste Care, another resident named Carl was frustrating to care for. Despite the many different approaches used with him, he seemed to be distressed and anxious most of the time.

CARL

Carl was admitted to the dementia unit several years prior to joining Namaste Care. When first admitted to the facility, he was able to walk and would occasionally join activities. As the disease progressed, he gradually began to have problems with falling and was deemed unsafe to walk on his own. He was evaluated by a physical therapist and, after breaking several wheelchairs, was given a special rocking wheelchair because he seemed to need to be constantly moving. Carl found a place in the corridor where he moved up and down throughout the day. He was resistive to care and from his expression seemed to be a very unhappy man.

The activity staff was unable to find anything that he enjoyed. Out of desperation, he was taken to the Namaste Care room, where he was placed in a lounge chair near the window. He seemed to be able to feel the sunlight and he responded to this peaceful setting by falling asleep. When agitated, he was spoken to in a soft voice; he liked hearing about activities that he had enjoyed in the past. One day when he became increasingly agitated, the Namaste carer knelt next to him and talked to him about his love of picking apples. His family had mentioned that this was one of his favorite activities each fall, and she used this as a way to honor his past. She gave him an item that provided the scent of apples and showed him pictures of apples. With a soft, soothing voice, she talked him through the ritual of apple picking; before long, Carl was asleep.

Nan was another surprise beneficiary of Namaste Care. All nursing facilities have residents who pace, and Nan was one of them. The staff finds it difficult if not impossible to get these individuals to rest. There is a difference between pacing and wandering. The resident who is wandering can usually be redirected and engaged by staff. The resident who paces has "places to go and things to do" and is not easily redirected.

NAN

Nan was a younger resident who had been on the dementia unit for several years. She had the most beautiful eyes and a smile that melted hearts, but she paced constantly. One day Nan found her way to the Namaste Care room. Perhaps it was the low lighting, the scent of lavender, and the soft soothing music and quiet atmosphere that called to her. Whenever she walked into the room, she headed for an empty chair, and for a few minutes she would look around the room before closing her eyes and going to sleep for 10 to 15 minutes. When she woke up, Namaste team members would offer Nan something to drink and some ice cream. Because of her constant pacing, she was at high risk for weight loss, so any calories the team could get her to consume were beneficial. So, for brief periods during the day, Nan appeared to welcome the peace of the Namaste Care room and was at rest.

The lesson in these cases is that if members believe that the life of any resident could be improved by Namaste Care, go for it! Maintain focus on the individual and how to help him or her to live more independently or happily.

As mentioned previously, the story of a resident named Matthew Wilk embodies the story of Namaste Care, as he was one of the first participants in the program. His story begins with how he was selected to receive Namaste Care.

Matthew's Story

Matthew was one of the first residents to participate in Namaste Care. He met the criteria for Namaste Care because he was no longer ambulatory and needed total care. At first he could still respond to yes-and-no questions and motion to pictures placed in front of him. Gradually he could only communicate with his eyes and lost all verbal communication. Matthew seemed to recognize his wife Celia, who visited often. Celia, like so many spouses, had tried valiantly to care for Matthew at home, at first on her own and then with adult day services. They had a wonderful marriage, as anyone could see from the light in Celia's eyes when she recalled their life together. Now, during the final months, it was increasingly difficult for Celia to visit. Matthew was slipping away, sleeping more than he was awake; it was difficult for him to respond to her words. Because he slept through the activity program on the dementia unit, he was taken to the Namaste Care room for the special individualized sensory programs. Celia enjoyed giving her husband hand massages and visiting with the Namaste carers and other spouses visiting their loved ones. Namaste Care provided both Matthew and Celia with a support group of caring people.

Matthew perfectly fit the criteria for Namaste Care. He received personalized care that identified him as a unique individual, and his personhood was not diminished in spite of the many losses he experienced because of his disease. His story shows how the philosophy and mission of Namaste Care can help those who are living with the disease maintain a life with moments of quality.

CHAPTER 3

Implementing Namaste Care

The implementation of Namaste Care begins with selling the program to the decision maker, usually the administrator, in your nursing facility. This is assuming that you, the reader, are not the decision maker. Request a meeting with the administrator in which you will be undisturbed, preferably away from a telephone. Offer this book, or information from it, prior to the meeting or as part of your presentation, and personalize the program to your facility. Use examples of real residents to show how Namaste Care will benefit the facility's residents. These touches help to make the program real, not a theoretical concept.

One administrator was swayed to advocate for Namaste Care by "the rabbi's" story. The rabbi, once a well known and respected member of the local religious community, was in the advanced stage of Alzheimer's disease (AD). This resident tugged on the heartstrings of the administrator and staff as they witnessed the toll that AD was taking on him. He looked so frail and lonely. Here is his story:

THE RABBI

His eyes were haunting. Most days the rabbi was in a lounge chair or in bed with a feeding tube that provided continuous nutrition. Often, a soap opera or the *Jerry Springer Show* was on the television set—the staff's choice, definitely not his. The rabbi was clearly well cared for, with clean clothes and his yarmulke firmly in place. He was in the advanced stage of AD, nonambulatory, and required total care; except for strong eye contact, he was nonverbal. The Rabbi rarely left his room because of his feeding tube. He did not participate in any activities other than occasional religious services, when he was wheeled into the room with his feeding tube equipment. Someone had to sit with him so that no other resident would touch the feeding tube. The activity department visited him several times each week and read passages from religious books, nursing took care of his physical needs, and occasionally he had a visitor. That left hours alone. What kind of quality of life was this for a man who had dedicated his life to others?

After checking with his physician, it was determined that he could go for periods of time without the feeding tube. Nursing staff members agreed that if he had a place to go, he could be taken off the feeding tube for these periods. In Namaste Care, the rabbi would not be alone. He would be with others and would benefit from those activities that were still meaningful to him. Namaste carers would talk to him, recalling his life's work that was so important to him and the community he served. He could listen to favorite religious music and chants that had been a major source of pleasure in his life. Music would be played for him on headphones or played for everyone in the Namaste Care room. The rabbi would be part of the Namaste Care community; he would be in the presence of others, as he had been throughout most of his life.

When the rabbi was taken to his room for tube feeding, Namaste Care would continue. Favorite music, as identified by his family, would be played or a video of religious services would be shown on his television. The cable would be disconnected and there would be no more soap operas or Jerry Springer.

Administrators want the best possible quality of life for their residents, but they also have fiscal responsibility for the facility. The next logical question from the administrator is usually, "How much will this cost?" Therefore, it is important to develop a budget that includes expenses and projected increase of revenue.

DEVELOPING A BUDGET

Staffing

The kiss of death for any proposed new program is to suggest that staff needs to be added. Adding staff to provide Namaste Care, at least in the beginning of the program, is not necessary. In most facilities, one care partner from the dementia unit is assigned to the Namaste Care room for the morning shift and one for the afternoon shift. During this time, other staff members can take responsibility for any of that care partner's residents as well as their own who are not in the Namaste Care room. Thus, the number of residents in the Namaste Care room is at least equal to one assignment for a care partner. Additional staff support for Namaste Care can come from a variety of departments; ask department directors to adjust shift assignments and be creative with budgeted hours. Here are a few examples:

- The activity director can change the location where activities are provided to residents with advanced dementia. Rather than going to each resident's room for individual visits, the visits can take place in the Namaste Care room. Having more staff in the room adds a sense of life and energy to the room and is more efficient for activity staff. If one resident is sleeping, an activity person can work with another resident. Activity staff can also gather two or three residents together.

- The activity professional for the dementia program or for the unit where Namaste Care is provided can be assigned to the Namaste Care room.

- Care partners and other staff on light duty can be assigned to the Namaste Care room.

- Hospice volunteers can be encouraged to use the Namaste Care room for visits.

- Facility volunteers can be recruited to work in the Namaste Care room.

Using this kind of creative staffing allows the program to be started quickly. Once started, Namaste Care has shown quick growth in most facilities and the ability to increase revenue. With increased revenue, hiring Namaste carers may be an option.

If the decision is made to add staff members, their hours are usually 9:00–5:00. The Namaste Care room is open from 9:30 A.M. until 11:30 A.M., or whenever lunch is served. It reopens at 1:00 P.M., or when residents have been fed and changed. The room closes at 4:30 P.M. The half hour prior to opening and after closing gives Namaste carers time to gather supplies and ready the room for their guests. It also allows time at the end of the day for charting and preparing the room for the next day. The Namaste Care program takes place 7 days per week. The salary that a Namaste carer receives should be higher than that of a care partner, activity assistant, or restorative aide. This provides an incentive for staff members to consider taking this position and gives them another career option.

Census Projections

Follow these steps to project how much additional revenue you can expect to receive from additional facility residents:

- Assess the existing dementia program and decide whether residents who no longer need the security of a dementia unit can be relocated to another unit where Namaste Care can be located. This would free up beds in the secured unit that could be filled with new admissions to the dementia program.

- Review the location of empty beds in the facility and decide if a dedicated Namaste Care wing would be a positive step in increasing census.

- Meet with local hospice programs to determine if offering Namaste Care would increase referrals from them.

- Visit referral sources and gauge whether offering Namaste Care would increase referrals to families looking for placement for a loved one with advanced dementia.

New programs often have a trickle-down effect. Even though a family might not need Namaste Care for their loved one upon admittance to a care facility, they may recognize the value of a facility offering such a program.

Physical Plant Costs

The Namaste Care room may be a space solely used for the program or a room that is shared and used for other purposes when the Namaste Care program is not opened. When it is a dedicated room, strive to give the room a warm, comforting look. It is amazing what a coat of paint and a wallpaper border can do to improve the look of a room. Some facilities start small, first locating their Namaste Care program in a vacant resident room or small conference room. When the administrator sees how many residents need the program, a larger space to accommodate more residents is usually found. Start-up expenses will differ depending on what is needed, but may include the following:

- Paint and wallpaper border
- Emergency call system for staff (e.g., a wall call bell, telephone, or hand-held device)
- Removal (or disabling) of any overhead paging systems
- Window coverings that filter direct sunlight
- Heating and cooling system that can maintain the room at a comfortable temperature for residents who are frail and usually cold
- Flooring that can be cleaned easily and does not have a high gloss
- Sink for hand washing
- Refrigerator
- Soap and towel dispensers
- Music system
- Television set with VCR and DVD capabilities
- Nursing supplies (see Appendix B)
- Quilts or coverings for residents

Remember to keep furnishings cozy and homelike. Furniture needs include:

- Locked cabinet for supplies

- Reclining lounge chairs (many residents will already have a wheelchair that reclines; hospice patients can get a lounge chair as part of the Medicare hospice benefit)
- Small tables (over-the-bed tables will work) for residents' personal items
- Chairs for visitors
- Storage for individual resident quilts and personal care items

Additional information on decorating the Namaste Care room can be found in Chapter 6. Lists of activity supplies, such as rain sticks and other sensory items, can be found in Appendix C. Sources for these supplies can be found in Appendix D.

Management Team

When the budget has been approved by the administrator and a green light given to go forward, the management team must be convinced to support the program. It is difficult if not impossible to start Namaste Care without their support. The entire management team needs to be knowledgeable about the Namaste Care concept, and their input must be requested and acknowledged.

The director of nursing (DON) is at the top of the list of people who must agree to the program in order for it to be successful. Namaste Care is primarily a nursing responsibility; in fact, DONs have called it an "enhanced" nursing program. The DON is responsible for Namaste Care. She selects who provides direct supervision of the program and ensures that all regulations and infection control issues are addressed.

Other key managers include the following: the activity director, who provides staffing hours as well as activity supplies and program ideas; the director of maintenance, who is responsible for making renovations to the Namaste Care room and ensuring that all equipment is in compliance with fire and safety codes; the director of housekeeping, who is responsible for keeping the Namaste Care room supplied with linen and maintaining the room in a clean and safe condition; the director of admissions, who is responsible for marketing the program, publicizing it to referral sources, and discussing Namaste Care with new admissions; and the social worker, who is responsible for helping family members understand how Namaste Care can provide quality of life programming for their loved one.

As part of the buy-in process, the administrator should schedule a meeting with all department managers to present the Namaste Care program. After the initial meeting to disseminate information and answer questions, the administrator and department managers should develop a plan for implementation.

IMPLEMENTATION PLAN

With the backing of the management team, the implementation process begins. Review the implementation plan often and change it as needed. A sample implementation schedule follows:

1. Schedule an information/education meeting with all staff to explain Namaste Care. This meeting may include educational information on dementia. Educating all staff employed in the facility about AD is one of the first steps in making sure that the facility is dementia friendly.

2. Insert a letter into staff paychecks explaining Namaste Care. Translate this letter into other languages as necessary.

3. Schedule a family meeting to explain Namaste Care and answer any questions.

4. Follow up this meeting with a letter to families and/or an article in the facility's newsletter.

5. Schedule a meeting with alert, oriented residents to discuss Namaste Care and answer their questions

6. Decide on the location of the Namaste Care room as well as the Reagan Room (a private room for actively dying residents; see Chapter 6).

7. Interview staff members who may want to work in the program.

8. Select and/or hire Namaste Care team members.

9. Issue a press release on Namaste Care.

10. Meet with local hospice programs and other referral agencies to explain the program.

11. Provide special education for the Namaste carers who will lead the program.

12. Purchase supplies.

13. Decorate the Namaste Care room.

14. Identify potential residents for the program and approach their families.

15. Determine a start date for services.

16. Schedule to have extra staff available on the opening day.

17. Plan an opening celebration; include all staff and referral sources.

After Namaste Care has been introduced, the energy surrounding it will carry the implementation through the challenges that always surface when starting something new in a nursing facility.

INTERNAL MARKETING

Internal marketing is highly important. It is a mistake to implement a new program or make major changes without letting all staff know what you are doing. Rumors begin flying, and misinformation is difficult to wipe away. There are many ways to let staff know as soon as the decision has been made to go forward with Namaste Care.

Introducing Namaste Care to Facility Staff

Informing all staff members in the facility, taking into account days off, sick days, and vacations, is a challenge. A mandatory meeting for all staff is recommended but may not be feasible because of the high cost of bringing in staff members when they are not scheduled to work. Also, many of the employees have two jobs or have child care responsibilities that make attending a special meeting outside of their shifts difficult if not impossible. An alternative is to schedule several short 30-minute meetings during a 2- or 3-day period. Assign one person to lead the meetings to provide consistency.

Even after this initial educational meeting, the person responsible for the orientation of new employees should integrate

Namaste Care information into ongoing staff education activities. Here are some creative ideas for staff education:

- Hold a special in-service and award a certificate to all those attending. Ring a chime or an Indian singing bowl to begin the meeting. The magical sound creates a dramatic beginning to the presentation. (See following section for an outline of this in-service.)

- Provide education during a working lunch for each department; serve food during the presentation and use the opportunity to personally thank all staff members for their participation.

- Pamper staff with Namaste Care supplies and activities. Give hand massages, play soothing music, and distribute lollipops to simulate some of the programming offered to residents during the Namaste Care day.

Outline of Staff In-Service

The following outline describes how information on Namaste Care, as well as AD, could be presented to the staff:

Introduction

A speaker, usually the administrator or director of nursing, introduces him- or herself and informs the staff of the purpose of the meeting. Staff members are provided with handouts that include a brief description of Namaste Care and the philosophy of the program.

Overview of AD

During this time, review basic information about AD, including symptoms, onset, risk factors, and stages; also discuss the benefits and burdens of cardiopulmonary resuscitation, hospitalization, treatment of infections, tube feeding, catheters, and medication.

Comfort Care

Spend time emphasizing the importance of comfort care for these residents. Explain to staff the Namaste Care philosophy on clothing, lounge chairs, bathing, and grooming.

Namaste Care

Finally, introduce the staff to the basics of Namaste Care, including meaning (Chapter 2), philosophy (Chapter 2), Namaste Care room (Chapter 6), Reagan Room (Chapter 6), a typical Namaste Care day (Chapter 5), after-death care (Chapter 9), examples of residents in your facility who would benefit from Namaste Care, staffing (Chapter 4), supervision, chain of command, weekends and shift changes, breaks and lunch, role of various departments, implementation, timeline for implementation, and staff selection (include instructions for interested staff members about whom to contact to schedule an interview).

The in-service usually lasts 45 minutes; allow another 15 minutes for questions and comments. Encourage participation by asking if the staff can see how Namaste Care would benefit particular residents. At the end of the in-service, give each staff member a lollipop, a Namaste Care hallmark.

All facility staff should be encouraged to spend some time in the Namaste Care room in order to understand the program. Often, care partners will learn from Namaste carers about a particular activity a resident enjoys, such as hand massages, and will try doing this special activity on their own when they have a break in the day or if the resident becomes agitated. Namaste Care techniques are helpful for all staff to use for calming residents.

Huddles

During the implementation process of Namaste Care, all involved team members should be provided updates on a regular basis. These updates offer an opportunity for Namaste carers and other staff to hear about the progress of the program as well as the next steps in the implementation process, and for administrators not only to squash any rumors but solicit questions and suggestions from the staff. This can also provide a forum to thank all team members involved for their help in making Namaste Care a reality. I call these sessions *huddles*—brief meetings scheduled at a time when most of the team members are present. Here are some good opportunities to call a huddle:

- Waiting for lunch to be delivered: No one is on break or at lunch; nurses and care partners are usually gathered in the dining room where residents are assembled waiting for the meal to be delivered and housekeeping and activity staff can join the group in the dining room

- During changes of shift

- During a large-scale resident entertainment program when most of the residents are occupied

- Any time that the nursing staff suggests; the staff has a better feel for what needs to be accomplished and when colleagues are taking breaks

After Namaste Care has started, huddles can be held in the Namaste Care room with all of the residents present. A care partner from another unit can keep an eye on residents during the huddle, or you may want to consider asking the administrator or other department manager to fill in for nursing staff during a huddle. This show of support from administration goes a long way in helping the care partners feel that Namaste Care is important.

Remember to keep meetings brief and avoid adding any extra pressure or tasks on care partners. Include night staff in some huddles. Although this staff does not work during the hours when the programming occurs, it is important for them to feel included and knowledgeable about Namaste Care. Keep huddles brief and positive. For any information that is not covered in a huddle, consider posting notices near the time clock; this ensures that all staff members will see the postings.

Huddles offer an opportunity for staff to discuss what is going well and what challenges are occurring. During these meetings, new ideas will be generated that will make Namaste Care grow and make your facility's program unique. Namaste Care is like a butterfly, and a facility's staff members give it wings.

Evaluation and Ongoing Communication

After Namaste Care has officially begun, evaluation and ongoing communication must occur on a regular basis. At least once a month, Namaste carers and other team members who work with the residents should have an opportunity to discuss the program. The team can be asked to recommend additional residents who would benefit from Namaste Care, keeping the program growing. Namaste carers should also review the status of current residents and share what they know about activities each resident enjoys.

Mechanisms should be in place so that any administrator or department manager can evaluate the program to assure its ongoing integrity. A Namaste Care checklist, for example, aids in this evaluation process (see Appendix E), assuring that routine maintenance procedures are followed and supplies kept on hand. Oversight by the administrator or department manager should occur on at least a monthly basis.

Introducing Namaste Care to Families

A special meeting should be scheduled to inform current family members about the plans to implement Namaste Care. They will begin to hear about it through the staff, so it is important to inform them as soon as possible after a decision has been made to implement the program. Family members, especially those who have a loved one with dementia, need to understand how Namaste Care is unique. If Namaste Care is going to be a dedicated wing in the facility, make it clear that when residents with dementia reach the advanced stage of their disease, the facility staff may recommend a transfer to the wing. Introducing Namaste Care to families provides the facility with an opportunity to educate family members on the medical issues that accompany the advanced stage of dementia. Inviting a health care expert, hospice provider, or the facility medical director to give the presentation or to conduct part of the meeting is also a good way to attract families to attend.

Families are often a good resource for attracting new residents. A happy family member is the facility's best spokesperson. One support group leader, the spouse of a man in the advanced stage of AD, went to a support meeting so excited about a new program offered at her husband's nursing facility. Rather than her usual tears, she enthusiastically spoke about Namaste Care and described the hand massage her husband was receiving when she visited. She described wanting to stay in the calming Namaste Care room instead of making her usual brief visit to her typically unresponsive husband. This testimonial enticed another family member who attended the meeting to transfer her husband to this facility.

Introducing Namaste Care to Residents

The alert, oriented residents in a nursing facility are well attuned to their surroundings and need to know the details of Namaste Care. The president of the Resident Council should be informed about Namaste Care and a special meeting should be scheduled for residents. At the meeting, residents should be told about Namaste Care, given written information on the program, and asked for their feedback.

Make the meeting enjoyable by demonstrating hand massages and offering lollipops or ice cream to everyone. Residents should be encouraged to visit the Namaste Care room when it opens. This is also a time to recruit resident volunteers who may be willing to sit with residents in the Namaste Care room.

This resident meeting provides an opportunity to open related discussions about hospice care or advanced directives. These are topics, it turns out, that residents find less distressing to discuss than their family members do. A woman named Mary, who was in a great deal of pain and approaching the end of her life according to the nurses, expressed a common sentiment when asked if she was afraid of dying. "Oh, no," she replied, "It's the living I fear!" Residents report that they do not want to die in pain or alone, and most are just amazed at having lived so long. The residents who attend the meeting about the Namaste Care program seem comforted to know that this type of program is available to them if they need it.

EXTERNAL MARKETING

Public Relations

Public relations and the marketing of Namaste Care to the local community should begin as soon as the decision has been made to implement the program. A press release is a good way to inform the media of this new program; include information about the program as well as a contact number. Press releases must be followed up, especially if the object is to get coverage for an event such as the opening of Namaste Care. Media sources need reminders for several days leading up to the event. When the program is in place, media outlets can be invited to view the program and interview Namaste Care team members.

Inviting the press to cover Namaste Care can be very positive, as long as you are well prepared. When the press is invited to the building, take measures to ensure that everything is sparkling. Remember that the overall impressions of the building, residents, staff, and care will influence the story that reporters write and the pictures they take. Prior to their visit, you may want to send written material or gently explain what they will encounter. Residents with advanced dementia can be shocking to those who are unprepared.

Remember to inform the staff in advance that media personnel will be in the building. You may want to schedule an additional care partner to help get residents up and groomed, looking their best that day. Each resident in Namaste Care should always be well groomed; on a day when the media is in the building, take extra care to have residents look their best. Housekeeping should also be advised and, if necessary, overstaffed in order to get the building in shape for the visitors. Take a walk outside the facility before the press arrives to make sure trash is picked up and landscaping is in good condition. I'll never forget one building I once toured. The dining room was nicely set with flowers on all of the tables, except the flowers were all dead. Many years later, I still remember the image.

The Namaste Care room should be set up with Namaste carers giving hand massages and providing sensory activities. When reporters see the activity in the room, witness the happy expressions of residents with lollipops in their mouths, hear the beautiful music, and smell the scent of lavender, they will have a positive image of Namaste Care.

Remember to obtain photograph release forms from families. Family members of Namaste Care residents may have strong feelings about having pictures taken of their loved one at this time of life. Inform photographers before they come to the facility about who they can and cannot photograph or film.

Giving interviews to the press is a great opportunity to tell the Namaste Care story. But remember that what gets printed is sometimes the impressions of the interviewer, not what the interviewee actually said. The person interviewed can ask to see a copy of the article before it is published, but this request is rarely granted. To avoid any surprises, prepare for an interview by developing a list of talking points. These are key responses to questions and what you want to communicate in the interview. Learn how to effectively develop talking points by watching a Sunday news program featuring a politician. They give five or six answers no matter what the question is.

Talking points for Namaste Care might include the following:

- The name of your facility

- The meaning of Namaste Care, "to honor the spirit within," as it relates to residents with advanced dementia

- The groundbreaking nature of the program

- The focus on providing improved quality-of-life programming for residents with advanced dementia

- The beauty of the Namaste Care room dedicated to the new program

- The special private room available for residents and families to be together at the end of a life

- The satisfaction of family members with Namaste Care and with the exceptional care their loved one is being provided

- The specially trained Namaste carer

The marketing staff can help draft these talking points or they can be developed with input from the management team. A practice interview may help staff members feel more comfortable. Following are some examples from my interviewing experiences. These show how to respond to an interviewer's harsh questions in order to establish your talking points and make the interview a positive experience.

Interviewer: I understand that there is a great deal of abuse in nursing homes.

Staff: We all deplore hearing about the few abuse stories that are in the news. Thank you for providing me with an opportunity to talk about Namaste Care, a new program at [nursing facility]. It is the first program for residents with advanced dementia in the city. We are proud of our reputation of providing excellent dementia care. Our newest program, Namaste Care, is another example of how we are constantly adding services to help our residents experience a high quality of life while they are with us.

Interviewer: I understand this program is for people with advanced dementia who don't respond and can't remember anything. How do you know it makes a difference at this stage of their lives?

Staff: Namaste Care means "to honor the spirit within," and we believe that every person has the right to excellent care in the presence of others throughout their lives. Not only does Namaste Care at [nursing facility] give residents this quality-of-life experience, but families tell us they feel a burden has been lifted when they walk into our beautiful Namaste Care room and see their loved one in a comfortable lounge chair, listening to beautiful music, receiving a hand massage, and sucking on a lollipop.

Interviewer: So much has been in the news about finding a cure for Alzheimer's disease, won't you lose a lot of money if a cure is found?

Staff: If a cure is found, we will be the first to celebrate. However, until that day arrives we will continue to provide excellent care for people with all stages of Alzheimer's disease. Namaste Care is a unique program in [city] to offer this type of care to residents with advanced dementia.

Most of the time, reporters are polite and the questions are fair. Even when questions seem leading, they can be turned around so that the facility comes across as caring and professional. I once did a call-in radio show. The very first caller told me that he had advised his family that he would kill himself if he was ever diagnosed with Alzheimer's disease. My reply was that receiving a diagnosis of any terminal disease is devastating (validating his feelings) and that now medications and lifestyle approaches may help to slow the disease process. New medications are getting approved on a regular basis (offering hope) and the cure is closer. Then, to show him the fun that is experienced by residents with dementia, I told him about a recent visit to the Namaste Care room from a kazoo band. I ended the call with an invitation to visit the facility and see for himself how people can live with the disease (extending hospitality) and thanked him for calling. Whew!

Most interviews are not this challenging and most interviewers are very professional. It is a good idea to ask the interviewer how much time has been allocated for the interview. Knowing the time limitations will help you prioritize what to say. Also ask if the interviewer has any personal experience with someone who has AD. Often, he or she has personal experience that can be related to the audience; this gives the interview a personal touch.

Television coverage is usually limited to a brief interview, so making sure you get talking points across is not easy. The interview is usually shown the same day it is filmed or the following day. Ask when it will be shown so that the show can be taped for marketing purposes. Tapes of any good news coverage, as well as newsprint articles, are a bonus to show during marketing events. After the coverage, be sure to send a thank-you note to the radio or television station or newspaper.

Referral Sources

Health care professionals who refer residents want the best care for their clients. When the decision is made to offer Namaste Care, marketing material should be developed for referral sources. Referral sources usually like the idea that the facility is providing something out of the ordinary and that the administration is willing to put money, time, and effort into enhancing the care given to residents. Marketing staff members appreciate having something new to talk about during their calls to referral agencies. Agencies that may appreciate information on Namaste Care include:

- All referral sources currently in the facility marketing database
- The local chapter of the Alzheimer's Association or other groups devoted to AD
- Alzheimer's support group leaders
- Area Agency on Aging
- Hospice programs
- Physicians
- Health maintenance organizations
- Senior referral agencies
- Hospital discharge planners

An effective way to publicize Namaste Care is to offer a continuing education unit (CEU) program. This is an effective way to get health care professionals to the facility. Programs such as Namaste Care that provide the latest research on end-of-life care provide interesting clinical information. It is very effective to schedule the program when Namaste Care is in place and to invite attendees to observe the program in small groups after the presentation.

Usually the marketing staff likes to provide small items to those attending the program. If possible, these gifts should be related to the presentation. For example, a Namaste Care gift bag could contain hand lotion, lavender sachets, chocolate, and lollipops. A door prize could be a service at a day spa or a music box like those used in the Namaste Care room. Food served may include smoothies or ice cream.

Implementing Namaste Care is a process that requires support from all staff. Helping the program reach as many residents as possible is an opportunity to educate the health care community and families who have loved ones with AD that quality of life is possible for nursing home residents with advanced dementia and that your facility is leading the way in providing this special end-of-life care.

Matthew's Story

Matthew's wife Celia was invited to a family meeting held to explain Namaste Care to family members. This meeting was facilitated by the Dementia Program Director, the charge nurse on the dementia unit, as well as the charge nurse from the new Namaste Care wing. They were able to answer questions from family members who were concerned that they would have to move their loved ones away from units where they were familiar with the staff and happy with the care and activities provided. During the meeting, Celia began to feel more comfortable that the excellent care would continue in the new wing and that Mary, the restorative aide who had started providing special activities for Matthew, would be scheduled 5 days per week on the new wing. Celia knew that Matthew's condition was deteriorating and that she would have to be prepared for a move to the new wing in the near future. This meeting gave her a positive feeling about the care her husband would receive on the new wing and she felt more comfortable after hearing the charge nurse talk about Namaste Care.

CHAPTER 4

The Namaste Care Team

Providing good Namaste Care requires selecting staff members who are able to work with residents who have terminal illnesses. Do not assume that current staff members will embrace Namaste Care, especially if it is part of an existing dementia program. In some dementia programs, residents who are in the advanced stage of their disease are transferred to another wing of the facility. Few residents, therefore, actually die on the dementia unit. Caring for residents in the moderate stages of dementia is quite different from caring for residents in the advanced or terminal stages of dementia and requires a hospice-like approach to care. This work is not for everyone. Nurses, care partners, housekeeping, and activity professionals should be selected only from those staff members who have expressed a desire to work with Namaste Care residents. As part of the introductory in-service that explains Namaste Care, staff members are asked to talk with their supervisor if they are interested in working on the unit. They are then interviewed by the person supervising Namaste Care. A questionnaire for interviewing staff can be found in Appendix F.

It is assumed that all residents in Namaste Care will die while in the facility and that participating staff members need to be comfortable on a unit where death is a frequent presence. This requires a special calling. One of the important goals of Namaste Care is providing a peaceful, pain-free, dignified death in the resident's home (i.e., the nursing facility), surrounded by family (both relatives and staff). In addition, residents in Namaste Care are usually unable to communicate. In other long-term care settings, many elderly residents live for years. They can talk to staff members, joke, say thank you, and show love. The residents receiving Namaste Care are usually unable to do any of this. Some staff members find this kind of care exhausting and unrewarding.

Housekeeping staff in the Namaste Care program may also have additional duties. The Namaste Care room is not a typical nursing facility room; it will be filled with items such as plants and quilts to make it look as homelike as possible. Remember, too, that housekeeping staff members become close to residents and may not all be comfortable working among those who are terminally ill.

Namaste Care activity professionals need to enjoy working with residents individually rather than in the typical groups. They will have responsibility for providing individual sensory programming in the Namaste Care room and making bedside visits in residents' rooms. They will be expected to suggest stimulating supplies and to develop new program approaches for residents with advanced dementia. In many respects, all of this is new to activity professionals and an area in which few resources are available. Activity professionals will also have some responsibility for maintaining the Namaste Care cart. Selecting Namaste Care team members who are excited by the possibilities offered by a new program will help to ensure its success.

SELECTING NAMASTE CARE TEAM MEMBERS

Nurses and care partners selected for Namaste Care must be willing to provide care as meaningful activities and understand that the process is more important than the task itself. This is a paradigm shift for nursing staff members. For example, rather than trying to give a resistant resident a shower or tub bath, the care partner gives a relaxing bed bath. It is sometimes difficult for nurses and care partners to change from a *task-oriented* approach to one more focused on *process*. They must be willing to make activities of daily living meaningful. Traditional care partners are used to being assigned a certain number of residents to dress, groom, bathe, change, and feed. The day shift aides are also expected to make beds, tidy the residents' rooms, and complete their assignments by the end of the shift. Added to this is the expectation that, in Namaste Care, they will talk to and spend quality time with residents.

Nurses' responsibilities include calling physicians, charting, providing treatments, distributing medications, and talking with families, among a variety of other jobs that arise as the day unfolds. The Namaste Care approach asks team members to spend more time with residents and leave the other tasks until after the residents have been provided care in an unhurried way. The supervising nurses must support the care partners as they shift their focus to this person-centered philosophy and show understanding when, for example, every bed is not made on schedule. Nurses must also be able to model care approaches and give a helping hand when needed.

Care partners who express a desire to work with Namaste Care residents are interviewed by the charge nurse to make sure they have the necessary clinical skills. The unit director, if that person is not a nurse, may be included in the interview. During the interview, staff members are informed of the expectations of Namaste Care and assured that if they do not want to work on the unit, they will be transferred to another unit without any negative repercussions. Interviews also provide an opportunity to ask staff members how they feel about their work. Many care partners have worked in long-term care for many years and may have lost the enthusiasm they once had for the job.

JOHN

John had been a care partner in the same facility for more than 15 years. During the interview, he pleaded with the charge nurse to let him work on the Namaste Care unit. He said, "I've forgotten why I started doing this work in the first place. I think Namaste Care will help me regain that feeling I used to have. At the end of the day, I can go home and feel good about what I have accomplished that day. Now, I go home exhausted and think of everything I didn't get to."

If Namaste Care is part of an existing dementia unit and a decision has been made to use existing staff members rather than hiring a Namaste Care specialist, all care partners should be asked if they are interested in being selected to work in the Namaste Care room as a Namaste carer. Not all care partners who have chosen to work in Namaste Care will enjoy being in the Namaste Care room providing daily programming. Beware, however, of making assumptions about which staff members are best suited to the program and which are not. Sometimes the most task-oriented person, whom you would never expect to enjoy Namaste Care, becomes transformed by the magic that happens in the Namaste Care room.

BETTY

Betty was one tough cookie. A robust woman, she towered over the other care partners. She was a very negative person and the first to find a problem with most changes. That Betty loved the residents was very apparent, but her approach focused on getting the task accomplished more than the process of doing it. She was very proud of the number of showers she could do and that her beds were generally made before the other aides'. She listened to the Namaste Care presentation with a dubious look on her face. She said she was a better care partner than the others and would do the job if she *had* to. The unit had residents in all stages of dementia, so the unit director assigned Betty to the residents in the moderate stage of dementia.

The unit director had not selected Betty to be one of the staff members assigned to work in the Namaste Care room for obvious reasons. The week after Namaste Care opened, a huddle was held to get feedback from the staff. Betty got on a roll and told management it was expecting too much from the overworked care partners. The 9:30 A.M. start time was unrealistic and having five residents in the program was, in her words, "crazy." Other staff members jumped on board and supported Betty. They wanted management to hire more staff, which wasn't a possibility at the beginning of the program.

One day, the staff person who had been selected to lead Namaste Care called in sick. Betty was asked to fill in for her. "Absolutely not," she declared. She had not been selected at the beginning of the program and she was perfectly happy taking care of the other residents. The unit director realized that Betty's strong reaction might be because she had not been selected in the first place and her feelings were hurt.

The unit director asked the director of nursing (DON) to let Betty know that she felt Betty could do a very good job because she knew how much Betty cared for her residents. Betty reluctantly agreed. The next day the miracle began.

Betty arrived to take over Namaste Care with a small tabletop water fountain and plastic music box. At 9:30 A.M., Betty had more residents in the room than ever before. The look on her face as she was providing foot massages was that of absolute pleasure. Everyone from the administrator to the DON visited Namaste Care that day to see the "Betty miracle." Namaste Care not only enhances the lives of residents, it can do wonders for staff morale and job satisfaction.

BIG DOUG

Affectionately referred to as Big Doug, this care partner was a gentle giant—a very tall, imposing figure but so gentle with the residents. During one particularly difficult time with staffing, Doug worked double shifts and appeared exhausted. Then, on top of everything, the Namaste carer called in sick and Doug was asked to fill in. As always, Doug agreed to do what he could and rose to the occasion beautifully. He had all of the residents looking comfortable in their chairs, music played, and a mood of tranquility permeated the room. As he gently bathed and massaged residents' feet, the exhaustion disappeared from his face. Another Namaste Care miracle.

Once staff members get hooked, they tend to stay with Namaste Care. Most find the work very satisfying and are proud when the staff from other units as well as health care professionals visit to bask in the peacefulness of the Namaste Care room.

SUPERVISION

Namaste Care is usually the responsibility of the DON because it is primarily a nursing program. The DON delegates the daily supervision to the charge nurse or the dementia unit director, who then assigns staff to lead the daily program and monitor the program to make certain it is being implemented properly. When the nurse responsible for the daily supervision of Namaste Care is not present, the unit charge nurse supervises the program. Sometimes, Namaste Care is supervised by the activity director. The Namaste Care checklist is a helpful tool for ongoing supervision and can be found in Appendix E.

Namaste Care supervisors are also responsible for helping Namaste carers and care partners feel appreciated. They have a difficult job, often a thankless one. Working day after day with residents who cannot carry on a conversation, say thank you, or remember their caregivers is not easy. Resident deaths are a fact of life, yet there is often little or no time to grieve. Families are another variable that may not always be easy to deal with. Some family members direct the frustration and anger evoked by the disease toward the nurses and direct-care staff. So, just as the residents need special care, so too do the staff members.

Verbal praise is an absolute must for members of the Namaste Care team. They should be greeted with the same respect and care with which they greet residents every day. Gestures such as hugging, if appropriate, asking about their families, and letting them know that the team is glad to have them back after a few days off, help them feel valued. Offering simple pleasantries makes such a difference. Fresh doughnuts or other goodies are a nice way to say thank you. When the supervisor does something personal, such as cooking something special for the team, the bond between team members is strengthened. Namaste Care is not only about a special way of caring for residents, it is about caring for all team members.

To reinforce this, a kind word from management, especially the administrator or DON, does wonders for team members' self-esteem. Timely evaluations, especially those that include a raise, show respect for staff members. Long-term care workers do not make a great deal of money, so even a small raise can make a difference to them.

Families often tell the charge nurse how happy they are with a care partner but do not tell the care partner. Family members should be asked to take the time to personally thank Namaste carers who do a particularly good job or have done something special for them or their loved one. Any written thank-you letter should be posted on the unit. If a staff person has been mentioned by name, the letter should be copied for the individual and the human resources director.

ASSIGNING SPECIFIC RESPONSIBILITIES

Namaste Care is usually led by a care partner, whose title is Namaste carer, with support from the activity department. The Namaste carer assigned for the day opens the Namaste Care room after breakfast and stays in the room until lunch. Other team members should come in periodically to relieve the Namaste carer for breaks and lunch. The Namaste carer may also assist with serving lunch to the residents on the unit.

After the residents have had lunch and been toileted, the Namaste Care room reopens. The afternoon program usually has fewer residents because some residents take a nap during this time. The Namaste carer assigned to the room may need to do charting before beginning afternoon activities. When the afternoon shift arrives, the Namaste carer is assigned to the Namaste Care room until the residents are taken to the dining area for dinner. The Namaste Care room could also be opened in the evening with one care partner in the room while the others are getting residents ready for bed.

Typical hours for the Namaste carer are 9:00 A.M. to 5:00 P.M. This leaves a half hour in the morning for gathering supplies and getting the room ready for the day, another half hour of quiet time before lunch to dispose of soiled laundry and refresh linens and other supplies, and a final half hour at the end of the day to work on charting and get the room ready for the next day.

HANDLING STAFFING SHORTAGES

Staffing shortages are a reality in the long-term care business, requiring supervisors to be resourceful. In these instances, it is more important to have the room open and staffed than it is to ensure that regular activities such as massages take place. Creative ways to staff Namaste Care in emergencies include the following:

- Ask each manager to volunteer to staff the Namaste Care room for 30 minutes. They can easily be given the proper education to do some of the meaningful activities or simply play music and talk to the residents.
- Ask the charge nurse to take a turn in staffing the room.
- Ask activity staff members to spend part of their day in the Namaste Care room.
- Ask administrative staff members, who are often nurses themselves, to volunteer for time in the Namaste Care room.

Another idea that adds extra hands in the Namaste Care room is to assign staff members who are on limited or light duty, who cannot carry out the tasks of their regular position yet have been released by their physician to return to work.

PATTY

Patty was a dedicated care partner who did not think Namaste Care was for her. She loved her work with the residents and the residents loved her. When her knee needed surgery, she was out of work for a month. Her physician gave her the go-ahead to work again, but ordered her to be off of her feet for the majority of the day—not realistic for a care partner who is on the go all day. The rehabilitation department ordered her a low chair on wheels, and she was assigned to help in the Namaste Care room. She fell in love with the program and, as they say, the rest is history.

TIM

Tim was a care partner who everyone dreaded having assigned to their unit. He had been around the unionized building and knew how far he could push the envelope without getting written up. He certainly had to know that the supervisors didn't like him and, as a result, became even more challenging to work with. One day when he was on light duty and planned to do as little as he could, the nursing supervisor assigned him to the Namaste Care room. Everyone held their breath waiting for him to explode with anger, his usual reaction when he didn't like something. To their surprise, Tim was inspired! He shaved the men, massaged feet, and joked with the ladies; the room shined! No one could believe it; one by one, managers trooped down to the Namaste Care room to see this transformation and congratulate Tim on doing a great job. Positive reinforcement made him glow. He said it was the best day he had experienced in many years. Namaste Care magic at work again.

RETAINING STAFF

The turnover of care partners in long-term care is more than 71% each year (Decker et al., 2006). For human resources, it is a never-ending cycle of recruitment and orientation; staff members work a few months and leave, and the process repeats itself. Attracting and retaining good staff is difficult. The Pioneer Network has found that nursing facilities who have embraced culture change have a significantly lower turnover rate than the national average. These facilities have eliminated overtime, decreased use of temporary agency staff, and lowered compensation costs. Administrators report that staff members feel better about their jobs and want to be a part of something fresh and new (Pioneer Network, 2006).

Namaste Care fits in with the culture change movement, as it is about person-directed care and the rights of residents to continue to be involved in life for as long as they live and to be honored and cared for in a respectful manner. The quality of life they experience extends to the staff members who care for them. Namaste Care team members truly believe that their jobs help to improve quality of life. Because all Namaste Care team members are involved in decision making as the program evolves, they feel empowered to suggest changes. When staff members feel as if they are valued, turnover is significantly reduced. The Namaste Care approach to selecting, educating, and valuing the team helps to maintain stable staff members who know their residents and will help make nursing homes feel like homes.

CHAPTER 5

The Namaste Care Day

Namaste Care encompasses many aspects of residents' lives. It is an around-the-clock way of providing care that uses comforting approaches and fills each resident's day with opportunities to engage in meaningful activities. The Namaste Care team interacts with residents throughout their waking hours and honors them as unique individuals. One resident's spouse described entering the Namaste Care unit as being "enveloped by a giant hug."

Each resident's day is filled with unplanned activities, those hundreds of interactions with staff members that provide the opportunity for Namaste Care team members to touch and talk with him or her. These are moments for Namaste carers and residents to experience meaningful connections. The residents react and participate at their own level of awareness with their eyes, words or sounds, and body movements. Namaste Care reframes the meaning and process of providing for activities of daily living (ADLs). These become more than getting dressed and groomed for the day and are an opportunity to share time together.

And so the Namaste Care day begins for residents with advanced dementia with a gentle awakening to the day. When words fail, Namaste carers find other creative ways to communicate. Sally

Callahan (2005) wrote lovingly of communicating with her mother, even when dementia had taken all language away. She says, "Somehow, together, we learned the language of eye hugs and heartspeak; through eye hugs and heartspeak we found a spiritual connection." She further commented on feeling that not only was her mother calmed by their spiritual connection, but she was calmed herself. So, with heartspeak and eye hugs, Namaste carers help residents greet the day.

MORNING CARE

A typical day in a nursing facility starts with the morning shift of care partners getting residents up, serving and feeding them breakfast, and getting them groomed. This is all accomplished in a relatively short period of time. On a good day, when all scheduled staff show up for work, the typical care partner is assigned from six to eight residents. When staffing is less than optimal, each care partner might have 10 residents. "Frantic" and "rushed" are how care partners often describe their mornings.

Imagine, for a moment, how residents with advanced dementia must feel when staff members are this harried. Without any way of knowing that it is indeed time to rise and shine, the constant commotion from highly energized staff must be frightening. Residents don't know where they are and what is expected of them. They may also feel hunger, are usually wet, and have not quite adjusted their sleepy body rhythms to waking up. By contrast, Namaste carers help the residents greet the day feeling safe and in the hands of a friend.

The Namaste Care morning begins with music—a soft, gentle beginning to each day. When Namaste Care is located on a separate unit, the sound of beautiful music or of birds chirping fills the air. The music is usually a classical piece, love songs from the forties, or nature sounds. Morning is a time of awakening, and the music should reflect that feeling. Music influences everyone on the unit. Namaste Care team members seem to slow down and approach their work with a lighter heart as beautiful music drifts through the wing.

Namaste carers always knock on the resident's door and identify themselves before entering the room. "Good morning, Mr. Black. I'm Carol, and I will help you get ready for breakfast." This is a simple but courteous way for staff members to enter a resident's room. When the resident appears to have heard the greeting and is beginning to wake up, a light touch lets the resident know that someone is there. Carly Hellen (1997) speaks of *caring touch.* Touch is primarily how we communicate with people who have lost their ability to understand verbal messages. We touch "hello" to let residents know we are there; we gently move parts of their bodies to dress them; and together with the sound of our voices, our facial expressions, and eye contact, we make waking up and getting ready for the day a less frightening experience. A man in the early stages of Alzheimer's disease (AD) described the typical daily experience in nursing facilities as "waking up in the middle of a movie and having no idea what has just occurred." With soft reassurances and a loving touch from Namaste carers, however, residents feel assured.

Some residents like the drapes opened early in the morning, while others prefer dim light. Avoid turning on the television. When the television is on, staff members tend to talk less to the resident. Off with television and on with conversation, even if it is one-sided.

It is a good strategy to explain to the resident what is going to happen next and how he or she can help. For instance, a care partner might say, "Mr. Black, I'm going to help you get out of these wet clothes. I think you'll feel so much better. Can you help me by turning over?" Throughout morning care rituals, such as brushing teeth, washing faces, and combing hair, the care partner should urge residents to participate, even if it is just by opening their mouths or holding the facecloth.

Care partners should praise residents' efforts to take part in their personal care. The intentional shift in terminology from *caregiver* to *care partner* identifies the need for the person on the receiving end of care to remain as independent as possible. Residents, even those with severe impairments, must be given the opportunity to participate as a partner in the care partner–resident relationship. Speaking in a low tone of voice and giving explicit directions throughout the care process will maintain a connection between the care partners. Saying, "John, I'm going to help you get dressed for breakfast. If you just give me a hug, I'll help you sit up" is a positive way to involve the resident. Choice and control are always a part of Namaste Care.

Most residents in Namaste Care have lost the ability to communicate verbally, so care partners should watch for their nonverbal signs. The resident may communicate with facial expressions, body language, and sounds. If a resident is unable to make recognizable choices, the Namaste carer continues to talk to the person saying, for example, how handsome the resident will look in his clean shirt or that a woman has very beautiful hair that shines when it is combed. A resident who resists dressing and becomes agitated is perhaps communicating a wish to be left alone. In this case, Namaste carers should respect this choice by doing as little care as possible, simply ensuring that the resident is in clean pajamas and slippers.

People with dementia have difficulty dealing with the world around them, but Namaste carers can make it easier for them by making sure that hearing aids are working properly, eyeglasses are clean, lighting is strong, and dentures fit. Unless the resident is clearly uncomfortable with wearing glasses, dentures, or hearing aids, these items should be maintained in good working order. Residents with advanced dementia should not be burdened with excess disabilities.

As the morning care ritual is unfolding, Namaste carers are continually assessing for any signs of pain. Pain assessment begins the moment a care partner walks in the door and continues with every interaction. Namaste carers learn to read body language by watching the residents' body movements and facial expressions and listening to the tone of their voices. If a care partner believes that a resident is in pain, he or she should report this to the nurse on the unit.

Often, resisting morning care can indicate physical or mental distress. Taking time to sit with and talk to the resident is time consuming for staff but a necessary part of Namaste Care. It is also important for Namaste carers to know each resident's life story so that their conversations include important people and events in the residents' lives. Care partners, in general, find incredibly creative ways to work with residents. Successful ones know how to "think out of the box" and be creative and flexible.

MOLLY

Molly was a difficult resident for the day staff, as she resisted most attempts to get her up and dressed peacefully. Molly had severe cognitive and physical impairments; in fact, Molly needed assistance with all personal care. In the morning, she was usually curled up in a tight ball of resistance and soaking wet. It was frustrating to care for her because all attempts to get Molly to cooperate with personal care were greeted by striking out and screaming at staff. She may have been frail and tiny, but she had a voice and strength that belied her diminutive size. No one wanted her on their assignment list, except for one care partner who was very successful in getting Molly up and dressed. She even coaxed smiles out of her.

The staff was desperate and called me for a consultation. A huddle was scheduled to brainstorm approaches that might work with Molly. When the one care partner said she had no problems with Molly, we all stared at her. What, we asked, was her secret? She very hesitantly told us that when she entered Molly's room, she knocked on the door, said "Good morning, Grandma," and kissed Molly on the cheek. The care partner had stumbled on calling Molly "Grandma" when she had told Molly one day that she reminded her of her own grandma. Molly had smiled, and her eyes had lit up. This "Good Morning, Grandma" greeting became part of their special relationship. After Molly was awake, the care partner would say that she was taking "Fluffy" (the cat who had been Molly's best friend for years) off the bed so she could eat her cat food. She pantomimed removing the cat from the bed, after which Molly was happy to cooperate with her morning care.

How did the care partner know about Fluffy, we asked? She replied that she had been as frustrated as the rest of her teammates, so when she saw family and friends visiting, she made it a point to find out all she could about Molly. They told her about Fluffy and the strong relationship between Molly and her cat. Molly's daughter remarked that her mother was very protective of her cat and had slept with Fluffy for years. It occurred to the assistant that Molly might be curled into a ball to cuddle the cat. In spite of her advanced dementia, Molly had a strong connection with memories of the cat. Once the cat was out of bed and happy, Molly was content to allow her "granddaughter" to help her get ready for the day.

Creatively finding approaches that work makes job responsibilities fun and less like work. It has been suggested that a new beatitude for nursing facility staff might look like this:

Blessed are the care partners
Who are flexible
For they shall not break!

Namaste Care Programming

Once breakfast has been served and the majority of residents fed and groomed, Namaste Care programming begins, usually around 9:30 A.M. The Namaste carer assigned to the Namaste Care room gathers supplies and readies the room to welcome the morning guests. This person communicates to other care partners about his or her involvement in opening the room so that other care partners will monitor those residents assigned to the Namaste carer who are not in the Namaste Care room. It can be helpful for the Namaste carer to make rounds of the unit—or wherever the residents are coming from—to let all staff know the room is opened. The Namaste carer can help with transporting residents to the Namaste Care room by returning to the room with one resident. As soon as any resident is in the room, the Namaste carer cannot leave the room unattended.

Preparing the Namaste Care Room

Beverages and food are gathered or the refrigerator is checked to make sure the supply of food for the day is adequate. Beverages might include fruit juices, liquid supplements, and water. Food items may consist of orange slices, crushed pineapple, soft cookies, puddings, and ice cream. All food items and beverages must be marked with the expiration date to meet regulations, and the items that are out of date must be removed from the room or the refrigerator as directed by the dietary department.

Ideally, Namaste Care rooms have refrigerators so that food and beverages can be stored safely. Someone must be responsible for regularly cleaning out the refrigerator. In some facilities, this is done by the dietary department. In other facilities, the Namaste carer is responsible for cleaning and maintaining the refrigerator according to regulations. State and federal regulations require a temperature chart to be filled in each day by the responsible staff person.

Namaste Care team members might transport and store some necessary items, such as facecloths, towels, sheets, or quilts, in a small laundry cart. Other items are always to be stocked in the Namaste Care room, including basins, lotion, soap, nail care items, music, and sensory and activity items. All supplies must be in place at the start of each day so that the Namaste carer does not have to leave the room once the program begins. For the safety of residents, the room is never to be left unattended when residents are present.

It is useful to post at the nursing station a checklist for opening the room. Occasionally, someone who usually does not work in the Namaste Care room will be asked to take over the program for the day. The checklist in Appendix E can be adapted and used for opening the Namaste Care room. A list of residents participating in the Namaste Care program should also be posted at the nursing station and in the assignment books because gathering residents and transporting them to the Namaste Care room is a team effort.

Opening the Namaste Care Room

After supplies, beverages, and food items are gathered, music is playing, lights are on, and draperies are opened, the Namaste carer opens the room for the day's guests. The Namaste Care room creates a special mood that is apparent to anyone entering it. Music, the scent of lavender, and inviting looks show how unique this program is within the nursing facility. Families, staff, and residents become quieter and more respectful in this space and everything slows down.

Each resident who enters the Namaste Care room should be greeted by name and touched in some gentle way. The morning greeting is individualized to suit the resident and the Namaste Care team member. Some care partners believe that showing physical affection in public is disrespectful. For them a handshake or a touch on the resident's arm feels comfortable. Other care partners feel comfortable giving a hug to residents. Welcoming each resident as a unique person is a way to honor the spirit within. Using a preferred name or title is one way to do this. For example, in one Namaste Care program, one of the residents is affectionately called "Gramps" while another, who had been a surgeon, is addressed as Doctor Smith.

All guests, family members, friends, and staff are made to feel welcomed in the Namaste Care room. All are encouraged to enter. The door may be closed to keep the noise level down, but a sign on the door saying "Welcome to Namaste Care, please come in!" gives the appropriate message to visitors. Having a room large enough to accommodate 12–15 residents in lounge chairs is optimal. However, any size room will suffice. If facilities were to wait for the proper size room to be available, very few programs would ever be started.

Getting Comfortable

All residents who enter the Namaste Care room should be gently placed in a comfortable seat. This might mean they are taken from a wheelchair and gently placed in a lounge chair or simply made more comfortable in their own chair. Two trained staff members are needed for transferring a resident from a wheelchair to a lounge chair. It is a good idea to ask a physical therapist to look at how residents are positioned, especially those with contractures or who are at high risk for skin problems. Residents in the advanced stage of dementia are usually losing weight and at risk of developing pressure ulcers. Making them comfortable in a soft lounge chair as opposed to sitting in a stiff wheelchair is good for the skin. Residents often fall asleep, so a reclining lounge chair is more comfortable for these little catnaps. If a resident is receiving hospice care, the hospice program may supply a lounge chair or reclining wheelchair.

Once each resident is settled in an appropriate chair, a quilt or some other covering is placed around them. Many Namaste Care participants seem to enjoy having a quilt tucked in under their chins. It is like infant swaddling and helps them to feel secure and warm. Several years ago at a conference, a nurse presented a poster session on decreasing agitation among people with dementia by tucking bed sheets around them at night; the same idea has been applied here. As people age, their metabolism changes. Many of these residents are cold, even in warm weather. It can be difficult for team members who are feeling very warm as they are taking care of residents all over the unit to understand how cold residents may be, but it is an important point to reinforce.

A variety of coverings can be used; twin-sized quilts are the most popular, as they are easy to wash, do not need to be ironed, and are comfortable and cozy. Washable afghans and twin-size blankets are also good choices. Twin sheets can be used during the warm summer months or for residents who tend to prefer a light covering. All coverings should be colorful—not institutional white. Colorful prints and soft colors invoke a warm look and help the Namaste Care room look more like a family room.

Each resident requires his or her own covering for infection control compliance. Each article must be kept clean and be stored for easy access. Consider the following options:

- Identify each covering with the resident's name using a laundry marking pen or name tag.

- Launder coverings only when soiled.

- Place each covering in a plastic bag marked with the resident's name.

- Place covering and other personal items in individual storage containers.

Seating Arrangements

Where each resident is placed in the room depends on the needs and interests of the resident and the size of the room. Some residents enjoy being grouped together so they feel the presence of each other. Other residents enjoy being close to a window to feel the sunlight or to watch the colors and the movement of the birds. Sometimes placement is a matter of practicality. When it is Mrs. Gold's day for a bath, she is placed so that she can be taken from the room without disrupting other residents.

Music

As anyone in the caregiving profession knows, music is a universal language. There is some evidence that even comatose patients respond to music. The area of the brain that responds to music is the last to be affected by AD (Cuddy & Duffin, 2005). Music helps create the calming, enveloping mood that permeates the Namaste Care room. Consider the following types of music to convey different kinds of moods:

- New Age music that is soft and soothing for quiet time
- Nature sounds—birds singing, waterfalls trickling, the echo of animals in the wild—for stimulating the senses during an activity
- Big-band sounds for range-of-motion exercises or to help awaken residents in the morning
- Broadway musicals such as *Oklahoma*, *The Sound of Music*, or *The King and I* will get toes tapping
- Love songs from Bing Crosby, Frank Sinatra, and Patty Page for the afternoon when spouses visit
- Classical music; Pachelbel's Canon is a popular piece for creating a restful feeling
- Cultural music, depending on the background of the residents (e.g., Jewish chants, Catholic and Protestant hymns, ethnic music)

Part of the adventure of Namaste Care is trying different approaches to comfort residents in the advanced stage of dementia. Morning music may be more upbeat to help everyone greet the day. Or perhaps a softer sound to ease the tension of the busy morning is more appropriate. The assistance of a music therapist can be helpful in selecting soundtracks to play.

A Scent of Morning

When the majority of residents are in the Namaste Care room, programming begins with orienting residents to the start of a new day. Providing a scent to harmonize with the weather and the season is a good way to accomplish this. Many stores provide a variety of scents in essential oils, which are expensive, or candles or sachets, which are quite inexpensive. If candles are used, the wicks need to be removed so they cannot be lighted. Pine scents and spices such as cinnamon evoke cold winter days. Spring scents may include flowers such as lily-of-the-valley, lilacs, and hyacinths. Summer brings the smell of fragrant roses, watermelon, and rain falling; when combined with the sounds of seagulls, these sensory items may reach long-ago memories of happy days on vacation at the shore. During the crisp fall months, the aroma of apples and cinnamon are appropriate. Ask volunteers to make oranges with cloves inserted in them to put in the room. So far, the smell of burning leaves has not been bottled, but hopefully someone will figure out how to produce that familiar scent. Long before regulations made it illegal to burn leaves in your backyard, this activity was a family tradition and a strong indication that fall had arrived.

The best scents are the real things. One Namaste carer kept the room filled with lilacs when they were in bloom. Another brought freshly cut grass during the summer months. Supplies for programming are as basic as the program itself. It is all about the fundamentals of life, and nature is one of them. The look of delight on the face of a resident who has just blown the seeds off of a dandelion is heartwarming.

The smell of bread baking is another wonderful morning scent. Consider purchasing a bread maker and easy-to-use mixes; as an added bonus, the residents may be able to eat the homemade bread.

Keeping fresh flowers in the room is always a welcome touch. Make sure, however, that no residents are allergic to the flowers. Consider purchasing African violets, which bloom year round. Or, talk to a local funeral home about delivering flowers after a funeral is over. Think of the beauty of the flowers as a final gift from a stranger who even in death can touch our lives. Taken apart and put in vases, they can fill the room with beauty and fragrance.

The Finishing Touches

Shaving

Although most grooming is usually completed before a resident is taken to the Namaste Care room, shaving men in the Namaste Care room can turn a basic ADL into a pleasurable activity and create an incredible sensory opportunity. Shaving must be done by a trained care partner or nurse according to regulations. The act of shaving in public could be viewed as a violation of privacy, so be sensitive. If the resident enjoys a special shave in the Namaste Care room, make sure it is noted in his care plan. Make this grooming task an enjoyable process by shaving the way men were shaved years ago. As you do, the scent of shaving cream will permeate the Namaste Care room, a welcome reminder of days gone by. When a resident is resistive to the process of shaving, discontinue the activity immediately.

EARL

> Earl was the lead care partner on the Namaste Care wing. On most days, he was responsible for shaving one particular resident who did not like to be shaved. Earl was a good care partner and used all of the correct approaches. The end result was that some days the resident was not shaved and sprouted bristles that look great on Tom Cruise but were upsetting to the resident's family. Other days, Earl won the battle by successfully dodging the resident's attempts to hit him. One day, Earl decided to try shaving in the Namaste Care room. He was pleasantly surprised to find that the resident actually smiled when he was shaved!

Although shaving is primarily a male necessity, facial hair on women also requires attention. Removing facial hair on women should be done in the privacy of their rooms or behind a screen in the Namaste Care room. Using a safety razor (which must be disposed of afterward), facial hair can usually be removed quickly and without any problems. Taking pride in how each resident looks shows respect for the residents and their families.

Moisturizing the Face

Skin becomes drier with age, and applying cold cream or moisturizer to female residents' faces after they are washed is a wonderful reminiscence activity. In particular, Pond's Cold Cream has an aroma that ladies appear to remember. Using a plastic spoon and medication dispensing cups, scoop the amount of cream needed for each woman to avoid any danger of cross-contamination. At the start of each day, every woman in the Namaste Care room should have her face washed with a wet, warm cloth (but not dried, in order to keep moisture on the skin) and face cream applied.

Make-Up

Applying make-up, such as light lipstick, may be a welcome activity; however, more extensive makeup might be appropriate only with residents who have been accustomed to using full make-up every day, like Eleanor.

ELEANOR

Eleanor was a model years ago. The family proudly showed pictures of her modeling the latest Paris fashions. Even when she was older, she loved dressing up and would never think about going out without full make-up. Actually, family members noticed the beginning of dementia when she started looking, in their words, bizarre. Eyebrow liner went every which way, far above or below eyebrows, and eye shadow was much too dark. Lipstick went beyond the lips, and her hair, once meticulously colored and maintained with a weekly trip to the beauty parlor, was uncombed on most days. It was apparent that Eleanor was forgetting beauty shop appointments, something she never would have done. As the disease progressed, she lost all ability to groom herself and did not seem to care anymore. It was devastating to the family to see their mother looking like this. Namaste Care recognized that the best way to honor Eleanor was to make time for special grooming and for dressing her in the beautiful clothing provided by the family. Eleanor once again regained the title of "beauty queen."

Hair Care

Most women and some men enjoy having their hair combed. In the advanced stage of dementia, beauty shop appointments are often dismissed as unnecessary and can even cause discomfort for the resident. We know that residents possess inner beauty, but it is also important to maintain their exterior beauty. Short hair is easier to groom; if a woman can tolerate it, consider permanents and hair coloring if that is her family's preference. One pleasing activity in the morning is to comb everyone's hair with gentle strokes. Most residents enjoy the attention. It is important to keep hair care items clearly labeled and separated for sanitary reasons.

DORIS

My own mother always told me that no matter what physical condition she was in, she wanted to be a "natural blond" until the day she died. As an only child, it was my responsibility to make sure that no one would be looking at her in the casket and see grey roots! Be assured that Doris at age 87 was a natural blond for her funeral. I'm sure no one suspected she colored her hair.

One day per week, Namaste Care can schedule a Beauty Day to simulate the services of a beauty shop. An activity team member can assist with soaking, cleaning, and filing fingernails (nail cutting must be done by a care partner or nurse). It is easier to keep finger-nails short and clean. A light nail polish can be used if the resident previously used nail polish, or simply buff nails to keep them shiny and healthy. Beauty Day is a meaningful activity for residents in Namaste Care. In one program, a Namaste carer used the Beauty Day to treat one resident to something very special.

SARA

Sara lovingly braided the long hair of a resident, Ann, who seemed to have progressed to the point of almost never responding to any kind of touch. When asked why she bothered to take time to do this when Ann did not seem to care if her hair was braided or not, Sara responded that she had seen a picture of Ann when she was younger and noticed how beautifully her hair was braided. Commenting on how little Sara found that she could do just for Ann, this became her way of showing respect and honor for this resident's natural beauty.

Hand Washing and Massage

All of the residents in Namaste Care have their hands washed and massaged in warm water every morning. Their individual basins are filled with warm, soapy water, and one at a time hands are placed in the water as the Namaste carer talks to the residents and massages their hand in the water. Residents' hands are then dried, and lotion is massaged on the hands and arms.

MICHELE

Michele is the DON in one of the facilities with a Namaste Care program. Her support was invaluable to implementing Namaste Care. One day when Michele came into the Namaste Care room, she noticed a resident with an anxious expression on her face and clenched fists. The Namaste carer who was responsible for the program that day told Michele that in spite of all she had tried with this resident, there was no getting her to relax so her hands could be washed.

Michele went into action! She took a basin of warm water and sat next to the resident. She spoke very softly to the woman and the resident gradually allowed her hands to be placed in the basin. Slowly, the woman opened her clenched fists and her face showed pleasure, all traces of anxiety disappeared. Michele took the face cloth, filled it with water, and wrung it out, making a small waterfall. At this, the resident broke into the most joyful smile and exclaimed, "This is wonderful!" One seemingly small moment, but that is what Namaste Care is all about, one human touching another.

Nourishment

Never underestimate the power of food. It represents care, politeness, giving, and receiving. Families focus on food. Can you remember when you were small and not feeling well, your worried mother hovered around the bed trying to tempt you with food? She would be so grateful when you would eat or drink something, anything! Offering food and beverages as a social ritual is ingrained into our very being. We greet people in our homes with an offer of food or drink. Socialization usually involves food and beverages.

As residents' cognitive impairments increase, their appetites decrease and eating problems are expected (Gillick & Mitchell, 2002). It is part of the natural progression of the disease. Weight loss and dehydration are almost always concerns in the advanced stage of the disease. The ability to feel hunger and thirst seems to disappear in advanced dementia. Although this is a normal, natural way for the body to prepare for this last part of the life journey, it is very troubling for families and may lead to infections and other health issues.

Each resident is unique, so rather than just accepting food refusal as normal for advanced dementia, it is good practice to assess any resident for depression who begins resisting food. Antidepressants and other medications may help to improve mood and appetite but may cause some burden to the resident. Medications may produce a dry mouth, constipation or diarrhea, and a range of other unpleasant symptoms. In Namaste Care, an effort is made to tempt residents with small offerings of sweet and easy-to-swallow food and beverages. In addition, the atmosphere in the Namaste Care room seems to stimulate appetites. Residents, until they begin to actively die, seem to be able to take in some liquids and food and appear to enjoy themselves while eating.

Occasionally, a resident will have problems with swallowing as the disease reaches its final stage. Namaste Care team members should watch for any swallowing problems. Observation is critical when residents have limited means to communicate verbally. When swallowing difficulties occur, it may be helpful to have a speech therapist, one who understands the Namaste Care concept of quality of life, evaluate the resident. Sometimes, a feeding tube is considered. For residents with advanced dementia, however, feeding tubes do not extend life and have many burdens. For more information on feeding tubes, see Chapter 7.

Registered dietitians, who are skilled in providing nutritional assessments, can recommend different textures of food or show how to thicken liquids to make swallowing easier. For safety reasons, Namaste Care team members should be informed about any residents who have swallowing difficulties. Any residents who may not swallow or who pouch food in their cheeks should sit upright as they are being fed to aid in the swallowing process.

In Namaste Care, food and liquids are offered by hand as a normal part of the day, several times in the morning and again in the afternoon. Nothing is offered right before a meal. Namaste carers might also try using covered sip cups or adult traveler mugs. Small amounts of liquid offered several times a day have great health benefits for the resident with advanced dementia.

Families love hearing that their loved one enjoyed some nourishment that day. Even better, ask families to offer refreshments during their visits. State regulations concerning feeding by untrained individuals usually do not include family members, and if the feeding is done in the Namaste Care room, a trained care partner is always available if needed. Families often welcome the chance to do something productive, such as helping their loved ones to eat. This meaningful activity can ease the difficulty and frustration of visits with someone who is no longer able to communicate.

Families and Namaste Care team members should practice offering food in a way that is gentle, kind, and respectful. Even if the resident does not seem to understand, he or she should be told that a delicious drink has been prepared. Place the resident's hands around the cup and encourage every sip taken. If it is difficult to rouse a resident, gently stroke his or her cheek while talking about drinking something. This gesture may stimulate the resident into taking nourishment.

Fruit

Fruits are a wonderful source of nourishment and hydration for residents with advanced dementia. Pineapple is appealing to some residents; it smells good and tastes good. Canned, crushed pineapple is easy to swallow, stimulates the saliva and digestive juices, and has a chemical effect on the mouth that aids good mouth hygiene. Orange slices also are enjoyed by many residents. First, hold the orange slice close to tempt the resident with the fruit's smell, then dribble a few drops on the person's lips, which can stimulate him or her to suck on the orange slice. Witness the pure delight!

SAM

Sam was a wisp of a man. Hardly eating or drinking, the DON once remarked that she thought Sam was alive because of the love surrounding him in Namaste Care. Care partners were so tender as they moved him from the chair to bed. It was as if they held a tiny sparrow in their hands. He had gentle but very aware eyes and almost no recognizable speech. Somehow it still seemed that he knew you were present for him. One day, I decided to give Sam a taste of orange. I approached him with a piece of orange and introduced myself. When the orange piece was near his nose, Sam immediately opened his eyes and the eyes said "yes!" I gave him a quarter slice and he sucked on the orange with such vigor that his strength surprised me. Then, he looked at me with such gratefulness and love that I was hooked. From that moment on, my visits to the facility always included Sam and an orange slice. I know it was special for him and provided moments for me that will forever remain in my mind.

Lollipops

Lollipops are a fun way to keep mouths hydrated. Most residents will not chew on them because they lack the teeth or the strength to bite down. As always, assessment and observation is important to prevent any problems. Residents usually respond positively when a Namaste carer says he or she has a lollipop for them. Their smiles brighten the room. Small lollipops are inexpensive and easy to suck. Family members usually smile too when they come into the Namaste Care room and find their loved one sucking on a lollipop.

Smoothies

Namaste Care rooms should have blenders to make smoothies. These mixtures of fruit and high-calorie liquid are easy to make and are beneficial for the resident who has not eaten any breakfast or who needs the extra calories. These delicious nourishments can be made at a moment's notice and in small amounts. Use high-calorie products such as food supplements or ice cream and nourishing products such as canned fruit.

Yogurt

Yogurt is a natural food that is easily swallowed and comes in a variety of flavors. Yogurt carries less danger of choking and aspirating than milk for residents who have difficulty swallowing. It also improves the microbes in the intestines. Yogurt can be purchased in small, individual servings.

Beverages

Offer residents juice, especially cranberry juice that contains acid that is useful in preventing urinary tract infections in women. Milk and buttermilk may add calories but are constipating. Ginger ale may be accepted as a comfort food. The sweetness is appealing, but the bubbles may be bothersome; leaving the bottle uncapped will decrease the number of bubbles but keep the taste intact. Serve beverages at room temperature rather than cold or with ice. If you feel a cold drink will be more tempting, use a flexible straw that reduces the shock of the cold liquid. Pour small amounts to eliminate throwing the leftover away. Nutritional supplements are used for residents when ordered by a physician, based on the recommendations of the dietitian. Whenever possible, use typical beverages.

The morning routine for the Namaste Care program is simple, yet, like a day at a great spa, it is a joyful beginning for residents, their families, and the Namaste Care team members.

Matthew's Story

Matthew began the day by being gently awakened by the care partner assigned to him. He was changed, dressed, and groomed while the care partner talked about Matthew's wife and children. After breakfast, Matthew was taken to the Namaste Care room, where lively "wake-up" music was playing. He was greeted by the Namaste carer, taken from his wheelchair, and placed in a comfortable lounge chair close to the window. Matthew expressed how much he liked looking at the mountains when he was still able to communicate, so placing him near the window was a way to honor his wishes. A quilt was tucked around him and small pillows were placed around him to ensure maximum comfort based on an evaluation done by the rehabilitation therapist for how best to position Matthew for comfort and safety. Next to Matthew was an over-the-bed table with pictures of his family: one of his children, one wedding picture, and one recent picture walking on the beach with his wife Celia.

During the morning activities, Matthew was gently awakened by the sound of a bird (from a stuffed bird that makes genuine bird calls) and by conversation from the Namaste carer about his interest in golf. His favorite bird was a pheasant because it made a call that sounded like his name. Celia particularly enjoyed making the little stuffed bird chirp "ma-coo"; she would laugh and hug her "ma-coo."

A special treat for Matthew was getting shaved in the Namaste Care room. His chair would be placed near the sink. The Namaste carer would greet him with a kiss on the cheek, then remark that he looked scruffy; he smiled. She told him that he was going to have a wonderful shave so that he would look handsome for his visit with Celia in the afternoon. After a barber cape was placed around his shoulders, the Namaste carer gently washed his face with a wet, warm face cloth and then placed a small, wet, warm towel on his face. The next step was to tell him about the shaving cream that was going to be smoothed on his face. She continued to talk to him as he was shaved. When finished, the Namaste carer washed his face to wipe off any remaining shaving cream. This was one of the most pleasurable experiences for Matthew; he really showed a positive reaction. Celia told us that as a business-man he was always well dressed and groomed in the morning, and that Matthew shaved every morning, even on the weekend. Although Mat-thew could not shave himself anymore, he was honored by keeping this ritual intact.

Matthew was not consuming enough calories during meals, so the Namaste Care team made sure he had high-calorie snacks and bever-ages throughout the day. Matthew was known to have a "sweet tooth," so he was often given a lollipop to suck on. He was taken to his room to be changed and then went to the dining room for lunch.

AFTERNOON ACTIVITIES

The Namaste Care room has afternoon activities planned each day, although some morning activities are appropriate throughout the day. Some residents will only be able to tolerate being out of bed for half days, so what is offered to them will be different from what is offered to the resident who is able to stay in the program all day.

Videos

The Namaste Care room re-opens after lunch, after the residents have been groomed and toileted. The room welcomes residents with music just as it did in the morning. Every resident is greeted and placed in a lounge chair or made comfortable in his or her in-dividual chair. A large-screen television plays a nature video. Rain-forest scenes are soothing after lunch when many residents are sleepy after the physical exertion of eating. The splashes of color and movement of waterfalls or animals seem to attract the attention of some residents.

Videos of fish, flowers, and the ocean are available at video stores as well as in activity supply catalogs. Resources for activity supplies are found in Appendix D.

In the afternoon, a shift change may occur and a new Namaste carer takes over responsibility for the afternoon programming. The new person arrives with great energy, ready to assume the many tasks. However, a boisterous greeting and loud voice do not fit with the serenity of the Namaste Care afternoon program. A bit of sensitivity education helps Namaste Care team members realize that they must enter the Namaste Care room as a breeze softly flutters in a window, changing the feel of a room but not adding to or detracting from the atmosphere.

Snoezelen

Made by a Dutch company for children with disabilities, Snoezelen multisensory stimulation products also seem to appeal to adults with dementia. Most popular is a light with a wheel that can make the room look like a giant lava lamp. This piece of equipment can be used in the Namaste Care room or be transported to a resident's room to provide sensory stimulation.

Soft, Fun, Furry, and Familiar

Each afternoon, the Namaste carer or activity professional visits with each resident using a variety of items to explore ways to connect with him or her. Different fabrics, such as cashmere, silk, velvet, and rabbit fur, stimulate reactions. Used clothing, such as evening gowns, usually produces smiles from the ladies; perhaps they are recalling their younger days when they went to dances dressed in their finest. Used prom dresses and wedding gowns are inexpensive when purchased at second-hand stores and no cost when donated. Tuxedos and leather jackets for the men provide opportunities for recalling special occasions. Hanging these supplies on a coat rack or draping them on a chair helps to give the room a warm, homey feel.

Some inexpensive and fun items that are simple but effective include colorful pinwheels, fans, puppets, colorful small balls, and even chattering fake teeth. Singing Santa Claus figures and dancing mounted fish always make residents smile. Stuffed animals usually produce smiles. Most people have had a pet sometime in their lives, so these life-like animals may remind them of their furry friends. If a resident does not like animals, he or she will let you know. Men seem to be soothed by and enjoy large dogs that are easier to hold. Women like cats and soft rabbits. Stuffed animals are sometimes effective in soothing a distressed resident. Some women are comforted by holding a baby. Namaste carers only use realistic dolls when no other item provides the comfort that a doll produces; whatever works, works.

Sports items including golf equipment, basketballs, baseballs, uniform jerseys, and pictures of famous sports figures may be enjoyable, depending on the resident's level of awareness and interests. Keep trying different items until one creates a positive response.

JOE

> According to his family, Joe was an avid Red Sox fan. Staff decided to reach Joe through his love of the game. When a baseball glove and ball, a Red Sox hat, and pictures of sports figures he had admired were placed on a table near him, he became a happy camper. He would smile and hold the baseball and glove, caressing the leather. Joe was basically unable to communicate, so imagine how surprised the Namaste Care team members were when he joined in a chorus of "Take Me Out to the Ball Game."

Even at the end of life, there is time for laughter. As previously mentioned, Matthew Wilk took his final breath as we were laughing about a funny story his wife had told. The charge nurse, his wife Celia, and I had been crying, and I guess Matthew decided that he couldn't leave such a sad bunch of women. We laughed, and off he went!

MARY

> The nurses had told me that Mary was dying. They did not expect her to live through the day. She was not responsive, but knowing that she was a very religious woman and being desperate to do something, I picked up the Bible and began to read it to her. Stumbling over words of places and names that were unfamiliar, a chuckle emanated from the bed. With a smile on her face, this dying resident said in a faint but clear voice, "You sure don't read the Bible much, do you?" And, with a smile still on her face, she drifted away.

Range of Motion

Residents involved in Namaste Care have lost the ability to exercise independently; they cannot follow directions and rarely move their hands and legs. In the afternoon, Namaste carers engage residents in passive range-of-motion exercises to provide touch, help prevent contractures, and get the blood circulating. A physical therapist should show care partners how to make this activity pleasant and beneficial for the residents. Passive range-of-motion exercise includes slow movement of the hands, fingers, arms, feet, and legs.

During range-of-motion activities, care partners must continually assess the resident's facial reactions and verbal sounds for signs of discomfort. This is one of those times when several pairs of hands can work wonders. Educate family members to do range-of-motion exercises, and encourage them to visit during this activity time. To make exercising more fun, play upbeat music. With the room filling with some big band sounds or a march, the residents are placed in a circle and the Namaste carers go from one resident to another providing range-of-motion stimulation and explaining what each procedure will involve. Even if a resident does not seem to understand what is being said, it is the Namaste Care way to explain every move to them.

Exercise can also be done with guided imagery. Tell a story and use a resident's arms and hands to describe the image. Say, "Let's look at how the sun is rising in the morning," and raise their arms as high as they will go without pain. Then talk about the breeze ruffling leaves in the trees and flutter the fingers. This is a very pleasant way to exercise.

Foot Washing and Massage

Readings of what is now known as hospice care contain excerpts from the journals of the knights of the round table. It seems that when they were too old to fight battles, they retired and were given the responsibility of caring for the oldest, sick knights. The description of how care was provided to the dying is as current today as it was hundreds of years ago. The writings spoke of providing clean linens, feeding warm soup, and washing the feet of the knights they cared for. There are also descriptions of Jesus washing the feet of the disciples. Foot washing is a humbling task and a loving gesture. In the Namaste Care room, foot washing is part of the day's ritual.

Foot massages are given using a careful and gentle touch, especially when rubbing over bony areas. Using a basin with soapy antibacterial warm water, the resident's feet are soaked one at a time, gently washed and dried, and massaged with lotion up to the knee. This procedure not only feels good but provides an opportunity for the Namaste carer to assess the integrity of the residents' skin and the condition of their toenails. Nursing is immediately informed of any questionable areas on the leg or foot. Toenails must be trimmed by a podiatrist, so except for the cleaning they are left alone. The reaction of residents to this very basic and loving experience is an expression of complete bliss.

Using Other Forms of Music

Namaste carers are amazed at the residents' reactions to sounds, such as the soft tinkling of a small wind chime. Dollar stores are good sources for these and also usually carry delightful little drums that make a soft beating sound. These items are easily visible, have motion, and make a pleasant sound. So many simple little objects are perfect for Namaste Care and well within the budget.

Rain sticks come in a variety of sizes and make beautiful soothing sounds; they can be found in most activity supply catalogs. Another stimulating instrument is the Indian singing bowl. It is more difficult to find but very interesting to use. The bowls make a humming sound that resonates throughout the room. Music boxes are so much fun, and residents usually recognize their songs and "tinkling" sound.

Another musical instrument is a QChord, which is like an autoharp but runs on batteries or by electricity (see Appendix D for purchasing information). Anyone can play it and make beautiful music. With assistance, even residents can strum the strings to produce beautiful sounds. There are also accompanying song cartridges that play a variety of tunes.

JOHN

> John was unable to participate in any activity program. Having just purchased a QChord, we were trying it on different residents. Namaste carers told me that John was a real challenge for them because he rarely reacted to any kind of stimuli. His wife told us that John had been a deeply religious man, so we played "Amazing Grace" on our QChord. As we sang the words, John started to move his lips and sing! His wife started to cry, as did all the team members around him. It was a deeply spiritual moment that occurred when music touched this man's life.

In the best of all possible worlds, employ the services of a music therapist once or twice per week. These are professionals who are very effective working in hospice and palliative care programs. Registered music therapists can be located through the yellow pages or on the web site www.musictherapy.com.

Recorded Tapes

Ask families to record messages on cassette tapes or CDs or, better yet, ask them to record the life history of their loved one. Residents will be happy to listen to these recordings again and again, perhaps reassured by the familiar voices (Camberg et al., 1999). After the resident has passed on, return the tape to the family with a sympathy card from the Namaste Care team members.

Nourishments

Nourishments such as the lollipops and juice are again offered in the afternoon. Make the afternoon special by also offering a treat such as soft ice cream or pudding. Some residents take pleasure in munching on a soft cookie that is easy to swallow and pleasurable to eat. Residents with advanced dementia usually retain a "sweet tooth," so anything sweet is usually enjoyable and provides much-needed calories.

IN-ROOM VISITS

If it is not possible for the resident to be taken to the Namaste Care room, then Namaste Care team members should provide in-room visits. Assemble a cart with the following materials:

- Lotions
- A variety of scents
- Sensory items such as realistic birds, a music box, pictures
- Soft fabrics
- A CD player and soothing music discs
- Hand wipes
- Plastic gloves
- Musical instruments
- A variety of reading materials (e.g., religious/spiritual, familiar poems)

If the services of a music therapist are available, schedule in-room visits. Entertainers and volunteers who play instruments that can be taken to residents' rooms may also be engaged to provide brief visits. A rolling cart with a television set and VCR or DVD player is also an excellent way to provide some comfort and stimulation for residents who must stay in their beds. Nature videos, musicals, and old television shows that the resident enjoyed may help the resident to feel less isolated.

If a resident is in bed for long periods of time and bed rails are used, cover the bed rails with soft material to encourage tactile exploration (Calkins, 2005). Placing soft stuffed animals in bed and long pillows on each side of the bed-bound resident may help him or her to feel secure and comforted. The important thing to remember is that Namaste Care is portable.

INVOLVING THE FAMILY

Most families visit in the afternoon. When their loved one is not able to speak and may not recognize them, visits are difficult. Many family members, especially spouses, visit almost every day and will look forward to having something to do. Their lives may be very empty with their husband or wife living apart from them. The visit not only helps them fulfill the commitment they made on their wedding day but gives them an opportunity for socialization with staff and other residents' families. Namaste Care team members become a close extended family when they show support to very lonely spouses. Some adult children also have a sense of responsibility to care for their parent and visit often. The Namaste Care room is the perfect setting for their visits.

With some assistance from staff, most of the materials used for Namaste Care activities can be used by families. Also encourage families to bring things from home that may elicit a response from the resident. Families are Namaste Care guests, so offering them something to eat or drink when offering beverages to their loved one is an appropriate and courteous gesture. Families enjoy seeing that staff members take such good care of the person they love.

Encourage families or visitors to take their loved one to a facility music program or for a walk (perhaps a stroll outside in their wheelchair). My grandson, Justin, was 6 or 7 years old when he visited his 103-year-old great-grandmother. He was so proud that he was allowed to push her in the wheelchair. Justin still treasures that memory. Just make sure that both the resident and family are in a safe situation when traveling out of the Namaste Care room. Many of the spouses are frail themselves and cannot manage wheelchairs without some assistance.

Matthew's Story

After lunch, Matthew was toileted and either put to bed or taken back to the Namaste Care room. Matthew was again warmly greeted by the Namaste carer. Many days he was not placed in a lounge chair because his wife was coming to visit and she wanted to be able to wheel his chair outside or be alone with him. To prepare for her visit, Matthew was told she would be visiting and a scarf with Celia's favorite perfume scent was placed around his neck. He loved Frank Sinatra and Dean Martin CDs, so he might have earphones with the songs he loved playing.

Celia arrived to hugs from care partners. They told her about Matthew's morning and all the positives they could communicate. As his condition deteriorated, it was important for her to hear that he was happy and well cared for. Like so many spouses, Celia had cared for Matthew for many years and it was difficult to turn his care over to others and to live without him. The Namaste carers were very affectionate and Celia had a healthy dose of hugs whenever she visited.

During the afternoon, Matthew had range-of-motion exercises. He seemed to enjoy a variety of musical sounds such as a rain stick, bells, or wind chimes. He especially liked chocolate pudding; his eyes glowed when the chocolate arrived and either Celia or the Namaste carer fed him.

Sometimes Namaste carers just held his hand and looked into his eyes. Matthew was loved and, with his peaceful demeanor, we believe he felt it. Namaste Care programming ended before the evening meal. Again Matthew was toileted and taken to the dining room, then readied for bed. Music he especially liked was played on a bedside tape deck. He was well cared for throughout the day with good nursing care and meaningful activities that enhanced his life.

And so the Namaste Care Room closes at the end of each day. Each resident guest is bid farewell with a touch. "Thank you for joining me this afternoon" and a hug are a perfect way to end the day for the resident and the staff. After the room is empty, the Namaste carer makes sure all soiled laundry is taken to the laundry room and the room is readied for the next morning by turning off appliances, wiping counters, checking food supplies, tossing out-of-date items, and so forth.

At the end of the day, the Namaste Care room is closed gently. I'm reminded of an old Girl Scout song we would end the day with, sung to the tune of "Taps":

Day is done, gone the sun
From the lakes, from the hills, from the sky.
All is well, safely rest.
God is nigh.

CHAPTER 6

The Namaste Care Environment

Namaste Care is offered in a variety of settings, depending on the space available in the facility. Each setting, in its own unique way, supports the program or services offered. The environment helps to shape the ambiance of the program, creating a sense of what takes place within its walls. This can easily be accomplished with the professional expertise of a designer; if that is not possible for budgetary reasons, there are numerous books available about designing environments for dementia care (Brawley, 2006). Couple these resources with a healthy dose of creativity from the Namaste Care team members.

In some facilities, the Namaste Care room is a vacant resident room. In other facilities, a large space is available. Some facilities designate a unit or a wing for Namaste Care. All spaces have challenges. Whether turning a resident's room into a noninstitutional space or making a large area look warm and cozy, Namaste Care team members must be resourceful and imaginative. It is important, however, to always remember that the essence of Namaste Care is not about the room itself but about a philosophy of care. Programming and special services can be offered anywhere that there is space to gather residents together in the presence of others. Whatever the allocation of space, small or large, giving it a different appearance from the rest of the building helps residents, their families, and staff members know that they are in a special place.

THE NAMASTE CARE ROOM

The Namaste Care room is a space designated for daily programming. It can be a room totally dedicated to the program or one that has several purposes. Ideally, a space is totally dedicated to Namaste Care programming and can be locked when not in use. In this case, it can be decorated with an array of antique objects, real plants, and other items that add warmth and character to the room. Several easy steps can guarantee a restful, cheerful environment.

The first step is deciding on the color of the room. Unless the room has recently been painted, repainting will give it a fresh, new look. Decide on the color scheme to use. Good choices include soft yellow, peach, green, or blue. Next, find a matching wallpaper border, preferably one with a floral print.

If getting the room painted would be difficult for the maintenance staff, recruit volunteers to paint and hang a border. Decorating the Namaste Care room is a perfect project for a service organization or generous benefactor. Painting and hanging the border is a one-weekend project with immediate results. Volunteers like to be able to make a visible difference. The Namaste Care room also provides an opportunity for fundraising. Some benefactors prefer to donate money rather than time and labor. Consider dedicating the Namaste Care room to the memory of a loved one of your biggest benefactor.

Once the room is decorated, the next step is to furnish it and add home-like touches. Here are some easy, affordable options:

- Look in facility storage closets and basements for pictures and furniture left behind by former residents.

- Visit Goodwill or used furniture stores for tables, cabinets, lamps, and other interesting pieces of furniture that will help to make the room look like a living room. Be on the lookout for buffets, as they are good storage pieces. Gently used furniture can be made more presentable with Old English polish that covers scratches. Stripping and staining old furniture is time consuming, but the finished piece can be a wonderful reminder of furniture that residents have owned in the past.

- Check out garage or yard sales for furniture.

- Purchase pictures and artwork at discount stores such as Wal-Mart or Target.

- Look for old items such as coffee mills, marbles, pieces of quilts, and bits of embroidery and lace.

- Ask for donations of plants or plant cuttings, and recruit a plant volunteer to keep them healthy. The local garden club may assist with filling the room with live plants and flowers.

- Repaint a bedroom wardrobe to use for storage.

- Hang wind chimes and brightly colored sun catchers in the windows.

- Ask families for pictures of the residents and arrange them around the room.

- Use doilies on tables to hide scratches and provide an old-fashioned look.

The simple placement of furniture and accessories can make a difference in how the room looks. For instance, adding a needlepoint pillow and afghan to a rocking chair placed beside a floor lamp creates a small, comfortable niche that family members gravitate toward. Likewise, couches are always popular, practical, and inviting. Before any electrical appliances are used, make sure that the maintenance department checks them for safety issues.

When Namaste Care team members have a vision for how the room should look, they often will find gems while shopping. In one facility, a rehabilitation aide discovered a buffet while she was browsing in a local Goodwill store. After it was polished and most of the scratches covered, it looked quite presentable. The drawers were kept open to show old lace tablecloths, colorful shawls, and other sensory items used for programming. It was a beautiful addition to the Namaste Care room. Old, used furniture pieces are perfect additions that help create a "lived in" look and, in some cases, are more inviting than expensive new purchases.

A Dual-Purpose Room

In some facilities, the Namaste Care room is used in the evening for alternate purposes. In this case, it is not feasible to equip the room with many of the home-like features of a room totally dedicated to Namaste Care, such as live plants, afghans on chairs, and antique items. It would be too difficult to keep these items in the room, especially in a dementia unit where residents may wander in and claim them as their own.

However, dual-purpose rooms can still look warm and friendly. Lounge chairs provide comfortable seating for ambulatory residents or those who are easily transferred from a wheelchair and can sit safely in them. A locked storage area is necessary if supplies are kept in the room; if this is not possible, a rolling cart with all of the supplies needed for the day can be taken out of the room when Namaste Care programming ends. Silk plants and flowers are used rather than live plants for residents' safety.

Although dual-purpose rooms are not the best option, you can always make do with what you have. Remember, the Namaste Care program usually expands quickly; as the population of residents with dementia grows, the possibility of creating a dedicated wing or unit becomes more viable.

Equipment

The Namaste Care room needs a sink, small refrigerator, and microwave. It is not difficult to create a kitchen area by hanging old kitchen utensils on the wall and placing old-fashioned magnets on the refrigerator. Antique dish towels, old-fashioned aprons on hooks, and a cookie jar help to fashion a country kitchen.

The biggest expense for many facilities is purchasing reclining lounge chairs, a comfortable alternative to wheelchairs. Found in long-term care supply catalogs, the lounge chairs look like what many people buy for their family room but they are made with different fabric. All furniture in a nursing facility must meet fire and safety regulations, so purchasing the chairs from a furniture store is not an option. Afghans on the backs of the chairs and needlepoint (looking) washable pillows make the chairs look inviting.

Another possible expense is purchasing a television with a VCR or DVD player. The television screen needs to be large enough for residents to be able to see the movement and colors. Nature videos with scenes from the rainforest or films of sunrises seem to catch their attention. The more alert residents enjoy watching videos of babies and pets; often residents smile as they view the shenanigans portrayed on the screen. Televisions also provide an opportunity for residents who are unable to attend religious services to worship. Catholic masses are often broadcast on Sundays, and Jewish services are available on video. These religious programs help meet the religious and spiritual needs of residents in Namaste Care.

The soothing, warm, cozy environment of the Namaste Care room enhances the programming. The room is also an effective way to create an identity for the program. The following example shows how one facility was able to implement Namaste Care quickly using the only available space on a dementia unit: an empty two-person resident room.

TRANSFORMING A RESIDENT ROOM

A resident room was painted the same color and had the same window treatments as all the other rooms on the unit. We wanted to create a different look yet not make any changes that would cause problems if the room needed to be reverted to a resident room. All of the furniture was removed and the room was painted a soft yellow. A flowered border was hung, and the room immediately began to spring to life.

The staff went on a hunting expedition in storage closets and in the basement. They found some small tables and paintings that had been donated to the facility by the families of deceased residents. An inexpensive plant rack painted a soft green was placed in one corner; it did not take up much space and added some color to the room. Families and residents donated their extra plants to the room, and we purchased an African violet for the window sill. These flowers are easy to care for and bloom most of the time. A bird feeder was attached to the outside window, providing enjoyment for several residents.

We discovered an old stereo system, the kind that looked like a piece of furniture popular in the seventies. It no longer worked and was not practical to fix, but we cleaned and polished it, and it became a useful piece of furniture. We covered it with a lace scarf, then arranged pictures, a basket of lollipops, and a plant on it. No one could recognize what it had been in its former life.

The room had two disconnected call bell units mounted on the wall, which made the room look institutional. An inexpensive patchwork quilt was purchased, sprayed with fire retardant spray, and hung over the fixtures with double-faced tape. The result was an inexpensive yet attractive way to hide the call bell system. Art for the walls and other interesting knickknacks came from the marketing department, which donated some items from the stash of decorating pieces used for model and respite rooms.

A private bathroom with a tub, toilet, and sink was already located in the room. Because no one was going to take a bath during Namaste Care, a pretty shower curtain was hung to hide a storage area for supplies created by placing a shelving unit in the bathtub. Residents would not be toileted in the room, so additional shelves were placed over the toilet. Pretty towels and a few pictures of old-fashioned bathrooms converted this resident bathroom into a practical yet pretty room.

Lounge chairs were not in the budget, but some unused geri-chairs were found in the basement. Their trays were removed, quilts were hung over the chairs, and cute pillows were placed on the seats to help hide the very institutional look of the chairs. In a few weeks and with little cost, this room was transformed.

It is amazing what can be done with great spirit and little money. It was fun to see the looks on the faces of staff and family members when they saw the transformation. If they only knew how we did it! Very quickly the room filled, and more residents than could be accommodated were identified as needing Namaste Care. Larger space was found so that the program could grow, and the original space was once again restored to a resident room. Using a resident room on a temporary basis meant that the beds did not have to be decertified, and the room with its new paint and border was desirable and quickly filled.

NAMASTE CARE UNIT OR WING

From a business perspective, designating a unit or a wing to Namaste Care has the potential to increase census. Prior to making this decision, a needs assessment is conducted. An evaluation of the current dementia program is a good first step. Assess the physical and cognitive status of the residents currently in the dementia program as well as residents on other units to determine the need for a dedicated advanced care unit. Then, determine the market for attracting residents with moderate dementia who would be needed to fill the beds of residents who would be transferred off the dementia unit.

Increased revenue from a special program is another financial consideration. Dementia units usually charge a higher daily rate than other units. Whether for-profit or not-for-profit, the reality of the health care business is that any facility must make money or at least break even. Most states are faced with the financial drain of their fast-growing Medicaid programs, and if they increase reimbursement, it is usually still below what it costs to run a nursing facility. Like it or not, the building has to make its profit on Medicare residents and by attracting privately paying residents. Revenue pays salaries, replaces furniture, and keeps the lights on. So, from a business perspective, making Namaste Care a profit center may be a good business decision.

From a quality-of-care perspective, a Namaste Care unit or wing can have its own dedicated staff, selected for the participants' desire to specialize in working with residents in the advanced stage of dementia. Staff members who choose to work in special units are usually extremely dedicated to their work and proud that they are part of a unique program. This was certainly true for the first Namaste Care program, which started as a dedicated wing in a skilled nursing facility in Bennington, Vermont.

VERMONT VETERANS HOME

The Vermont Veterans Home (VVH) in Bennington, Vermont, shows how a dedicated Namaste Care wing can be successful in many ways. From a business standpoint, it increased census by freeing beds on the dementia wing. Residents with advanced dementia were moved to an adjoining Namaste Care wing. The facility also experienced an increase in referrals from discharge planners and hospice staff who were working with families who had loved ones with advanced dementia.

Surveyors loved Namaste Care. They even asked permission to recommend that other nursing facilities in the state visit VVH to learn how to improve care for residents with advanced dementia. The unit also generated positive publicity for the facility in the United States, Asia, and Australia through presentations at conferences. Several articles were published on this Namaste Care wing.

The wing is part of a 17-bed unit divided by a central nurse's station. Fire doors are at the entrance to the wing, and the wing has the typical double-loaded corridor found in many nursing facilities. The Namaste Care room is located at the end of the corridor. The unit had one private room; the remaining rooms were for double occupancy. The social worker's office was located on the unit, as was a utility room and shower area with toilets. There was no budget for decorating the wing, so costs had to be kept low.

The institutional look of the corridor was changed by painting it a soft taupe and hanging a border. Walls were transformed with artwork from the local community. The facility initiated a "Gifts of Love" program intended to encourage local artists to donate original works of art for the wing. A letter describing the program and asking for donations (Appendix G) was sent to previous benefactors, artists, and anyone else who might contribute to funding Namaste Care. The letter was also published in the local newspaper as a public relations initiative. Several artists donated work; other benefactors donated money, which enabled management to purchase an adjustable double bed, bed linens, and carpeting for the private room. One of the VVH staff members was an artist, and she helped to group pictures and other decorative items on the walls, including the Chinese symbols for peace and tranquility, a small quilt, and pictures of the local landscape. The corridor was transformed from an institutional-looking space to one that was warm and peaceful—no easy feat with a very limited budget. When it was finished, Namaste Care team members found ways to disguise laundry carts and other unsightly items. They took great pride in how the wing looked.

Regulations require the name of each resident to be posted outside his or her room, so VVH staff purchased bulletin boards in a soft taupe fabric that had ribbons to hold memorabilia as well as the resident's name and room number. These were sprayed with flame retardant to satisfy fire regulations. Families were asked to provide copies (not originals) of pictures, as well as greeting cards or items that reflected the residents' past interests. One family tucked the resident's favorite recipe cards on her bulletin board. In this facility, all of the men and some of the women were veterans, so each bulletin board had an insignia showing the branch of service under which they had served. Small flags were tucked in the ribbons. Using bulletin boards that were beautiful yet practical made the long corridor come to life.

In this unit, fire doors were closed (but not secured) to lower the noise level. Soft music played in the corridor throughout the day. One team member was designated the lead care partner and assumed responsibility for turning on the music and ensuring that one care partner was always on the wing. Doors were kept open while residents were transported to the dining area and at night.

A shower room was located on the wing. It, too, received a makeover. Painting it blue, hanging pretty shower curtains and crisp white curtains, placing silk flowers on the window sills, and hanging old-fashioned bathroom pictures helped to make the room pretty. With all of the changes on this wing, anyone entering the doors knew immediately that it was a special place.

ADDITIONAL DEDICATED NAMASTE CARE SPACES

As the Bennington Namaste Care wing began to expand, team members began to look at all of the spaces on the wing to see how they could be used for Namaste Care.

Family Room

The social worker's office was on the Namaste Care wing, but she readily agreed to move so that a family room could be created. A donation paid for a sleep sofa for families who wished to stay overnight. Another family donated antique furniture that made the room look like an old-fashioned living room. A small table and chairs were added so that the room could be used for care plan meetings for the residents on the wing. Family conferences were held in the room, and families also used it for private visits.

The Reagan Room

Because residents who are actively dying and their family members need privacy, the administrator and board of directors approved the use of the only private room on the Namaste Care wing for that purpose. It was named the Reagan Room, in memory of former president Ronald Reagan, and its impact was fast and remarkable. Families were so grateful to have this private space to use during such a difficult time that they began to give donations to the Reagan Room. Many also asked their friends and family members to give donations in lieu of flowers in memory of their loved one. So the room was an instant success in many ways.

Families whose loved one was actively dying were given the choice of letting the resident stay in his or her room or move to the Reagan Room. Families on the Namaste Care wing were given priority, but the room was also offered to families whose loved one lived anywhere in the facility. Most families chose to have their loved one moved because of the privacy it afforded the family. We worried that it would be viewed as the death room. However, this was not the case, perhaps because we decorated it to look beautiful and because of the positive reactions from staff and families.

Inside the Reagan Room

The room was painted a soft peach, carpeting was laid, and blinds were hung on the large window. Donations allowed for the purchase of a dresser and a motorized double bed. This allowed Namaste carers to give care easily and spouses to lie next to their loved one as they were dying. Beautiful bedding was purchased for the bed. Two quilted bedspreads (so that one could be laundered while the other was being used), matching pillow shams, and peach-colored sheets and pillowcases helped to create a very home-like bedroom.

If you work in a nursing facility, you know that lost laundry is unfortunately a reality. Staff cringed when we showed them the beautiful linens we purchased for the room. They thought they would be laundered to death or disappear. That was never a problem because we went directly to the laundry department and asked for help. We explained about the Reagan Room and invited them to visit. We showed the laundry staff the bedding we had purchased and asked them how we could keep track of the items and keep them looking beautiful. They suggested personalized marking and gave us a special laundry bag for the items in this room. They seemed proud of their contribution to the room. We also met with the housekeeping staff. After explaining the room's purpose and our need to keep it ready at a moment's notice, they took special pride in polishing the furniture and keeping the room clean and in good order.

As soon as a resident was moved to the room, we transferred their mementos, pictures, and various other personal items. A box of items such as silk flowers and pictures for the bureau were gathered to keep the room looking personal even when it was unoccupied.

A reclining lounge chair ensured that families could be comfortable if they were sitting in the room or wanted to sleep. The Reagan Room had its own bathroom, which was painted and decorated with a pretty wallpaper border, matching shower curtains, towels, face cloths, bathmat, and wastebasket. Pictures were hung, and this formerly boring beige room was transformed to an attractive bathroom for families. Medical supplies were hidden from sight behind the shower curtain, so it was a practical space also.

The Reagan Room continues to provide a beautiful place for families of residents who are dying. The double bed was one of the best decisions we made, as it has made such a difference for families spending their last hours with a loved one. Joan, the wife of one resident, tells the story of her last night together with her husband.

JOAN

Joan received a telephone call one evening from the charge nurse. Her husband Jeffery was not doing well and she might like to come to the facility. She dressed quickly and drove to the facility as fast as she could. Joan had been living with her husband's AD for many years and, although she recognized that he was declining, she just didn't believe he was dying. He had a cold, but surely would recover as he had so many times in the past. When she arrived at the facility and saw Jeffery, she realized that his condition was more serious than she originally thought. The charge nurse took her to the family room and told her that she may want to call the rest of the family, as Jeffery's condition was quite serious. Joan was offered the use of the Reagan Room. She broke down in tears and struggled with the decision to move Jeffery. With gentle prodding from the charge nurse, she agreed to try it. He could always be moved back to his room if he got better. Joan says it was the best decision she could have made. For the remainder of the night, she lay next to Jeffery and held him in her arms. She talked to him about their life together and recalled memories from the day they met. As the sun was rising, she finished her story and Jeffery slipped away. Joan feels that somehow Jeffery heard her, and the closeness offered by the double bed made the passing an intimate experience.

Staff members have commented on how a special aura permeates the Reagan Room. Since the Reagan Room opened, it has created a haven for families.

Matthew's Story

Matthew was one of the first residents to be moved to the Namaste Care wing. Although it was a difficult decision for his wife Celia to leave staff that she had grown close to, she was grateful that his room would be close to the Namaste Care room. He was in the Namaste Care wing when his physical condition worsened.

Matthew was identified by nursing as entering the actively dying stage 4 days before his death. He was difficult to rouse, very lethargic, and developed a fever. The charge nurse called the physician, who agreed that comfort care should be continued and the fever treated with acetaminophen. The charge nurse and unit director approached Celia to see if she would feel comfortable moving Matthew to the Reagan Room. She had been watching the changes in the room and loved what had been created, so she agreed to have her husband moved. Matthew's personal pictures and other mementoes were also moved to the room. Music selected by Celia filled the room, and she decided that Matthew would enjoy having the drapes opened because he always enjoyed seeing the beauty of nature. Namaste Care team members checked on Matthew several times each hour to assess his condition, take care of his personal needs, and make sure Celia had food and beverages available and that she was comfortable being alone with Matthew.

He was kept comfortable with morphine and appeared to be very peaceful. Matthew's children arrived shortly after he was moved to the

Reagan Room, so Celia always had at least one family member with her. The family was offered food and beverages and overnight accommodations in the facility's guest room. When Matthew seemed to rally on the third day, his children returned to their homes in Massachusetts. As soon as they left, his condition worsened; it appeared that Matthew did not want to die with his children present. The Namaste Care team then stepped in to provide support and comfort for Celia. She was never alone for the last hours of Matthew's life. In the privacy of the Reagan Room, Celia was able to face the death of her beloved husband with a few chosen staff members who were with her until Matthew took his last breath.

Namaste Care is about providing special programming and offering unique services to residents with advanced dementia and their families. All can take place in a variety of spaces. The areas dedicated to Namaste Care should be as quiet as possible with no overhead paging or other institutional sounds. Call bells may be changed to produce a chime sound or play a tune to support the homelike environment of the unit or the room (Calkins, 2005). It is amazing how making the spaces comfortable and homelike and reducing the noise level can help to create a calming atmosphere. Namaste Care happens through Namaste Care team members' dedication and willingness to go the extra mile to make the dream of providing top-quality, compassionate care to their dying residents a reality.

CHAPTER 7

Difficult Decisions

Namaste Care is for residents with advanced dementia, a stage at which family members and physicians may be considering a shift in the goals of care for the resident from life at all costs to quality of life. From the time their loved one begins to show signs of dementia, family members are faced with a multitude of medical and psychosocial decisions that become more complex as the disease progresses. For many families, especially couples, facing the possible diagnosis of Alzheimer's disease (AD) is too frightening to comprehend, so they ignore or rationalize the signs of dementia. Most seniors are well aware that no cure exists. Even when diagnosed with an irreversible dementia, some families choose not to tell their loved one. However, this denies the person with dementia the opportunity to make decisions about care, including end-of-life care, at a point when he or she is still able to make decisions. Perhaps even more important, everyone has the right to know their medical condition.

Individuals in the early stages of dementia can make decisions regarding finances, designate a power of attorney, and participate in writing advanced directives and living wills. Taking these legal steps will help to ensure that wishes will be honored. The family and physician should initiate discussions about potential medical decisions as soon as the diagnosis is made. When the person with dementia is involved in planning for end-of-life-care, some of the burden felt by family members as the disease progresses is lifted.

In *The Best Friends Approach to Alzheimer's Care*, authors Virginia Bell and David Troxel (2003) offer the "Alzheimer's Disease Bill of Rights" (see Appendix H). The first right is that "every person diagnosed with Alzheimer's disease or a related disorder deserves to be informed of one's diagnosis." When the person does not want to hear or face the news, he or she usually just ignores it; most want to know.

The following situation occurred in a nursing facility and shows how adaptable residents are to receiving the diagnosis of AD.

MICHAEL

> Michael had been having problems with memory for several years. When he became lost while driving home his family took him to a physician who, after conducting a series of tests, diagnosed Michael with probable AD. His family refused to allow the doctor to tell Michael what was wrong with him for fear he would become depressed. When he fell and broke his hip, the family decided he was no longer safe at home and admitted him to a nursing facility. He was then also having trouble remembering names, even those of his grandchildren. Michael was becoming more and more distressed because he did not know what was happening to him. He kept asking the social worker what was wrong with him and then forgetting that he had asked, so he returned to her office to ask her again and again and again. She was of course not authorized to speak of his diagnosis. Eventually, she scheduled a meeting with the family members to discuss their father's right to know about the diagnosis. They reluctantly agreed to let him speak with his physician. A private meeting was set up in the social worker's office. When the physician explained that he believed Michael was in the beginning stage of AD, Michael replied, "Thank God. I thought I was going crazy. I can handle Alzheimer's disease; after all, President Reagan did."

LEGAL INCOMPETENCE

Each state determines the procedures for declaring a person legally incompetent. A person must be declared incompetent by a court of law, which will also appoint a power of attorney (POA). This is sometimes a long and expensive process. Until a POA is appointed, the resident is legally in charge of his or her own decisions—an unrealistic task for individuals with advanced dementia.

Decisions regarding end-of-life care are usually made with input from the attending physician, family members, and nursing facility staff. At times, however, disagreements arise between family members with regard to care and treatment decisions, and nursing facility staff may feel caught in the middle. Nursing facilities, especially those that offer Namaste Care, should make sure that a POA is designated for all residents. This will help to avoid complications.

Resources

Planning for end-of-life care can be overwhelming, but there are resources readily available. More than 11,000 web sites provide guidance on drafting living wills, which must be specifically designed for individual states. All states have some type of ombudsman program, which advocates for people living in residential long-term care settings and can help residents and families with a variety of issues, including referring families to organizations that offer legal assistance. If a resident is eligible for hospice care, hospice staff will provide assistance to families regarding end-of-life decision making. Hospice also offers grief and bereavement counseling for up to a year after the death. More about the Medicare hospice benefit can be found in Appendix A.

EARLY DISCUSSIONS REGARDING END-OF-LIFE ISSUES

Decision making is a process. In the early stages of AD, the goal may be to prolong life; as the disease reaches the end stages, the goal of care may be to provide comfort care. The social worker in the nursing facility should begin discussions with family members and, whenever possible, with the resident shortly after admission, once everyone has adjusted to the move. If the resident is able to take part in these discussions, some of the burden felt by family members associated with decision making is eased. Unfortunately, by the time many residents are admitted to a nursing facility, they are unable to participate in these discussions because they can no longer comprehend the issues.

Ideally, when a resident is admitted to a nursing facility, a POA has been designated and a living will is in place and/or the responsible party is clear about the wishes of the resident. Many residents and their family members, however, have not had conversations regarding end-of-life decisions and may still be in denial that AD is a terminal illness. In that case, decisions will continue to be made informally, without legal sanction, by the family and physician.

Unfortunately, problems can and do erupt when the family has no advanced directives to follow and family members disagree on medical decisions. The death in 2005 of Terri Schiavo, a young Florida woman who was comatose and did not leave written advanced directives, threw the United States into a fierce debate over end-of-life decisions. This emotionally charged case went to the floor of the Senate and eventually to the Supreme Court. The public battle pitted Terri's husband and parents against each other in the bright spotlight of the media. If advanced directives or a living will had been written, none of this heartbreaking trauma would have occurred. On a positive note, as a result of this case, more Americans now have signed living wills than at any other point in history.

THE NURSING FACILITY'S RESPONSIBILITY

The federal Patient Self-Determination Act (PSDA, P.L. 101-508, 1990) requires nursing facilities that participate in Medicare or Medicaid programs to provide residents and their families with written policies on advanced directives. On admission, residents and their families are given copies of these policies and must sign that they received them. Each person's medical record must include information on the resident's advanced directives, if they exist. Namaste Care offers personal attention and meaningful activities even when it has been decided that the person will no longer receive any medical interventions. Namaste Care nursing and social work staff members can help family members make difficult decisions by providing education on the burdens and benefits of medical interventions.

Care Plans

The interdisciplinary care team can schedule care plan meetings to help make families aware of the potential medical issues that are associated with AD and other dementias and to help them make decisions about the goals of care. Usually the goal for most residents in Namaste Care is to provide comfort care. Care plan meetings are held on a regular basis according to federal and state regulations and whenever a significant change of condition is noted. The facility must inform family members of the date and time of the conference and place a copy of the letter in the resident's medical record. If the family does not attend the meeting, someone on the care planning team should call the family to discuss the care plan or be sure to review the plan during the family's visits.

Namaste Care team members should attempt to involve as many family members as possible in the discussion of the care plan and goals of care so that the family understands and supports the interdisciplinary team. Some options for getting families to meetings include the following:

- Schedule meetings when the majority of family members can attend.

- Involve family members who are unable to come to the facility by using telephone conference calling.

- Be flexible enough to schedule a meeting on the weekend if that is the only time the majority of family members can attend.

- Use e-mail to connect with family members, making sure that privacy regulations are met.

Meetings with families help to build strong connections with department managers and Namaste Care team members. Schedule enough time for the meetings so that family members can talk about their feelings and so that team members have an opportunity to discuss decisions that may have to be made in the future. This will give the family time to consider the various treatment issues.

MEDICAL DECISIONS

The following information is based on studies regarding nursing facility residents with advanced dementia and supports the Namaste Care philosophy of comfort care as the primary goal.

Cardiopulmonary Resuscitation

Initiating cardiopulmonary resuscitation (CPR) on a resident with advanced dementia has enormous burdens and is rarely successful (Zweig, 1997). The numerous complications include fractured ribs, admission to a hospital's intensive care unit (ICU), and placement on a mechanical respirator. The ICU is especially frightening to those with dementia, and most admitted to the ICU will need to be sedated. Studies show that of 114 nursing facility residents who were admitted to a hospital after CPR, only 10% were discharged; the rest died in the hospital (Ghusan, Teasdale, Pepe, & Ginger, 1995).

Hospitalization

Hospitalizing a nursing facility resident with advanced dementia is also ill-advised. Unless the resident absolutely cannot be treated comfortably in the nursing facility, a transfer to an acute care center often results in decline of the ability to transfer, increased risk of decubitus ulcers, and loss of weight (Volicer, McKee, & Hewitt, 2001). Many residents who are hospitalized return to the nursing facility with in-dwelling catheters and on significantly more medications.

From the moment the ambulance crew arrives, the nursing facility resident with advanced dementia is plunged into a world that is alien and terrifying. Upon arrival at the hospital, the resident usually spends time in the emergency room. A variety of tests, confusing and occasionally painful, terrify the resident who cannot comprehend the reason for these procedures. More often than not, the resident is then transported back to the facility. If admitted to the hospital, the resident's anxiety intensifies.

Acute care staff members are not as familiar with the needs of patients with advanced dementia as nursing facility staff are. People with advanced dementia are unable to understand that they cannot get out of bed without assistance and do not comprehend the purpose of items such as catheters and IV tubes; many times, they must be restrained or sedated in order to keep these interventions in place. Pressure ulcers are a danger for frail residents who are restrained in their beds for long periods of time. Residents with advanced dementia need to be hand fed and coaxed into eating, a time-consuming task for nurses. They also require offers of liquid several times per day because they are not able to pour and drink.

Many residents return from the hospital on increased medications. In order to manage confused or distressed behavior from the resident in the hospital, he or she may be given antipsychotics or benzodiazepines, sometimes both. The resident may also be given medication to aid sleeping. All of these medications can produce dry mouth, constipation, and lethargy, among other unpleasant conditions.

Once in the acute care setting, residents experience unpleasant medical interventions such as blood tests, X-rays, and CT scans. When considering whether to hospitalize a resident, the burdens and benefits of these procedures must be weighed. Will the resident's life be more comfortable as a result of the hospitalization? It is important to remember, and to remind families, that orders can be changed at any time. For example, if a resident breaks her hip, her family must decide whether to surgically repair the hip of the resident who has not walked for some time and probably will not walk again. In this case, consider the fact that the hip will heal on its own with bed rest and appropriate pain medication. The resident may rest comfortably in her own familiar bed or in a reclining chair in the Namaste Care room among staff members who understand her needs.

Tube Feeding

Almost all individuals with advanced dementia in Asia are restrained in hospitals and tube fed. The Chinese have a saying that it is better to be "a fat ghost than a thin one," so tube feeding is the accepted treatment for anyone who will not eat or has swallowing difficulties. In the United States, decisions regarding tube feeding seem to be very emotionally charged. Before deciding to insert a tube, the pros and cons of this procedure must be considered.

There is evidence that feeding either with a nasogastric (NG) tube or through a percutaneous endoscopic gastrostomy (PEG) tube does not increase survival rates of individuals with advanced dementia. Research also indicates that tube feeding does not prevent aspiration pneumonia and may actually increase its risk (Finucane, Christmas, & Travis, 1999). The belief that tube feeding will lower the risk of pressure ulcers and decrease the risk of infection has been disproved in studies. The procedure to insert a feeding tube is uncomfortable and can be expensive.

An NG tube can be inserted by a nurse. Because NG tubes are uncomfortable, residents with them are often restrained or have mitts placed on their hands so they will not pull out the tube. In a study of patients who were alert and oriented and who had recovered from a stay in the ICU, results showed that tube feeding was the most uncomfortable procedure that the patients encountered, more uncomfortable than being attached to a ventilator. Being restrained was third on the list of uncomfortable procedures (Morrison et al., 1998).

A PEG tube must be inserted by a specialty physician and requires hospitalization. Evaluation for a PEG tube insertion requires consultation with a speech therapist to document that food is entering the lungs, as well as the services of an X-ray technician and radiologist to determine swallowing capabilities. This test requires swallowing barium, something the resident with advanced dementia may not be able to do. Inserting PEG tubes is a surgical operation requiring anesthetic. As with any surgery, there are risks inherent with the procedure, including infection and increased confusion from the anesthetic.

Consider antidepressant medications as an alternative to tube feeding for those residents who can still swallow but have stopped eating. Almost all residents in Namaste Care can be tempted with small amounts of preferred food, such as orange slices and lollipops. The enjoyment of food may be one of the last pleasures that residents with advanced dementia have.

The following story about Nathan and his mother Julia is one example of how a son was able to feel comfortable about keeping his mother in the nursing facility rather than hospitalizing her for hydration therapy.

JULIA

Nathan was recently divorced and retired and had little to do except focus on caring for his mother, Julia. He visited every day. Clearly, he was devoted to her and was stricken with grief that she was in the last stage of dementia. Julia slept most of the time and getting her to eat or drink anything was a miracle. During his visits, usually at lunch, Nathan would become either elated that she ate or drank something or very frustrated when she refused all attempts to feed her. He often had her hospitalized for hydration therapy when she refused to eat and drink. Nathan told me that he felt he had to do something; he could not let his mother starve. His mother's physician discouraged him from having a tube inserted but did agree to hospitalize her for hydration therapy.

The day Namaste Care began, Julia was sleeping in her wheelchair. When I approached her to say hello, I observed black-and-blue marks all over her arms. Alarmed, I was informed by the staff that Julia had once again spent a few days in the hospital for IV therapy. The places where the needles had been inserted and where the restraints had been secured were bruised. Julia pulled out the IV without the restraints, but her skin was fragile and tore easily. Even a small amount of pressure could cause skin discoloration and abrasions. It was heartbreaking to see this tiny little woman looking as if she had been in a prize fight and lost.

Julia was moved from her wheelchair into a reclining lounge chair, and a soft quilt was tucked around her. Small pillows were positioned under her arms, and a lollipop was offered to her. She opened her eyes and smiled when she tasted the sweetness and she sucked greedily on it. We had our first success story. Her son arrived shortly after the room opened and panicked when he could not find his mother in her usual place in the day room. The staff led him to the Namaste Care room, where soft music was playing, the scent of lavender was in the air, and his mother, very comfortable in the lounge chair, was sucking on her lollipop, eyes opened and twinkling with delight.

Nathan started to cry. Now, I panicked. What had we done wrong? He said it had just been so long since he had seen his mother so happy and comfortable. He began to tell me how awful he felt seeing his mother in the hospital, about the ambulance ride, painful testing, and the restraints needed to keep his mother from pulling out the IV. We talked about how very difficult it was for him to let go of his mother. He asked if she could be in Namaste Care every day. When told yes, he went to the nurse's station and informed them not to hospitalize her any more. He could see how comfortable his mother was and wanted her to stay with the staff that knew and loved her. She died a few weeks later, and he said that he was at peace knowing that her last days were spent in the arms of Namaste Care.

Treatment of Infections

Every nursing facility has infection control procedures that must be followed. Infections are the most common complication for people with advanced dementia. Respiratory infections and urinary tract infections (UTIs) are the most common of these. Although infections are routinely treated in the early stages of the disease when the person still has years of a quality-of-life existence, at some point in the advanced stage of the disease the family and physician should discuss whether antibiotics should still be used. If comfort is the main concern, then over-the-counter pain medication and morphine may be the treatments of choice.

Pneumonia is a common infection. Studies reveal that the residents with advanced dementia are as likely to survive the episode while treated in the nursing facility as being treated in the hospital (Fried, Gillick, & Lipsitz, 1995). Urinary tract infections can be also treated with comfort measures in the nursing facility.

Residents with advanced dementia are unable to report early symptoms and sometimes will not run a fever, one of the easiest ways to identify infections. By the time they do show signs of infection, its severity can make curing it difficult. If antibiotics are to be used, a diagnostic work-up needs to be made. This could involve blood tests, X-rays, catheterization, or other uncomfortable procedures.

All of these diagnostic procedures should be explained to the family members so that they can make an informed decision. Antibiotics also have side effects such as nausea and diarrhea (including *C. difficile* infections) that need to be considered for the comfort of the person. Many times, the resident can be made comfortable, and the simplest treatment may be the best.

JAMES

James was clearly in the advanced stage of dementia. He had almost stopped eating and drinking. He weighed less than 100 pounds. All of his needs were being met by staff; he was unable to speak, needed total care in his activities of daily living, was nonambulatory, and could only be out of bed for short periods of time as he was at high risk for skin breakdown. He began to show signs of a respiratory illness, probably pneumonia the nurses thought. The physician ordered X-rays, and James was treated with antibiotics and given an oxygen mask. In spite of his frailty, James made it very clear that he did not want that mask on his face. His small hands pulled and tugged at it until he was able to get it off. James was definitely communicating his discomfort. The Namaste Care nurse assessed his behavior and evaluated the effectiveness of the uncomfortable mask. The physician agreed that comfort was the goal and discontinued the order for oxygen. James went back to bed and went peacefully to sleep. He survived pneumonia on his terms.

Namaste carers are always listening to and watching residents who communicate with body language when verbal communication is no longer possible.

Nursing Procedures

Good nursing practice and nursing facility regulations require certain nursing tasks such as weighing residents, monitoring blood pressure readings, taking temperatures, and measuring pulse and respiration rates. However, some of these procedures may be changed for the comfort of the resident with advanced dementia. Following physician orders and federal and state regulations, the number of times these tasks are done may be altered. Taking weights, for instance, may be unnecessary when the family and physician decide not to use tube feeding or any other intervention when a resident is refusing food. Instead, the resident's upper arm or thigh could be measured, a more comfortable procedure than weighing. If the decision of the physician and family is to change routine nursing procedures, the resident's care plan must be altered.

Medication

Medications may have some side effects that are unpleasant. At a certain point in the life of a resident with advanced dementia, medication for chronic conditions may be discontinued or modified, as it will no longer be useful. Vitamins and medications for lowering cholesterol levels or for slowing the progression of AD have limited effectiveness and are not indicated at this time unless they are used for the comfort of the resident. Medications for discomfort from arthritis or joint pain as well as other medications used for the comfort of the resident are always indicated, as the comfort of the resident is the goal of care.

QUALITY OF LIFE, NOT LIFE AT ALL COSTS

Decisions regarding care options for nursing facility residents are ongoing throughout the disease process. When a palliative or comfort care approach is used, it sometimes appears that care is being decreased. Namaste Care shows families that their loved ones are receiving more specialized services and more activities that are meaningful at this stage of residents' lives. Quality of life is the focus. The emphasis is not on the number of days left in a person's life but on the quality of those days. Namaste Care honors each resident, surrounding each with a loving environment and in the presence of others.

Matthew's Story

Matthew's family chose to discontinue hospitalization and not to pursue tube feeding when he no longer wanted to eat. Celia and the Namaste carers could tempt Matthew with sweet stuff that produced looks of pleasure on his face. They recognized that the end was near and decided to keep him comfortable and avoid aggressive medical interventions. Celia and Matthew's family wanted him to die as he had lived, with dignity and surrounded by people he loved.

CHAPTER 8

Comfort Care

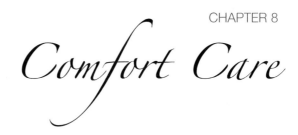

One of the primary goals of Namaste Care is to provide comfort in all aspects of life for residents with advanced dementia. The term *comfort care* usually means not using aggressive medical interventions such as hospitalization, tube feeding, blood tests, and other uncomfortable or confusing diagnostic procedures. Namaste Care believes that comfort care measures include the following:

- Managing pain and discomfort so that each resident is comfortable around the clock

- Offering activities of daily living (ADLs), which include dressing, grooming, oral care, toileting, feeding, bathing, and ambulation, as meaningful activities

- Clothing residents for comfort

- Providing a comfortable environment

PAIN

Alzheimer's disease (AD) does not cause physical pain, yet many residents with AD experience untreated pain from other medical conditions such as cancer, fractures, arthritis, tooth decay, osteoporosis, and other conditions. Pain is often undertreated or not treated at all because residents with advanced dementia have lost the ability to communicate. Undiagnosed pain occurs in 26%–83% of nursing facility residents and is a significant problem (Huffman & Kunik, 2000). Residents with dementia depend on staff to recognize when they are in pain and to provide relief. Therefore, residents must be continually evaluated for pain and discomfort by the Namaste Care team.

Namaste care partners and nurses are usually the first to recognize discomfort; however, all staff members are expected to report behaviors that may be signs of pain. This includes the Namaste carer assigned to the Namaste Care room, who spends long periods of time with the residents, as well as housekeeping staff.

Namaste Care believes in the hospice philosophy regarding pain: Believe the resident. If the resident is able to communicate and says or acts as if he or she is in pain, then it is treated. Without adequate pain management, residents in pain cannot experience a quality of life. Any attempt by the Namaste carer to provide meaningful activities will be difficult if not impossible. In order to make quality of life a reality, recognizing, assessing, treating, and monitoring pain in residents with advanced dementia is crucial.

Recognizing the level and location of pain in a resident with advanced dementia is like solving a puzzle; Namaste carers must uncover the clues. Residents may show the following signs that they are in pain:

- Facial expressions that show discomfort, such as grimaces, frown lines, and tense expressions
- Tension in the body; stiffness; unwillingness to respond to a request to move
- Less independence in performing ADLs
- Noisy, labored, or rapid breathing
- Shrinking or wincing when touched
- Rubbing a part of the body
- Avoiding the use of a part of the body
- Curling into a fetal position
- Decreased range of motion
- Keeping eyes closed

A resident in pain may sound like this:

- Saying, "It hurts"
- Saying, "No!"
- Screaming
- Swearing
- Moaning
- Crying or whimpering
- Changing vocalization or tone
- Making repetitive sounds

A resident in pain may behave like this:

- Resists transferring to a wheelchair
- Fights attempts of staff to perform ADLs
- Grabs staff
- Refuses to eat
- Appears restless
- Acts agitated
- Does not engage in preferred activities
- Exhibits problems sleeping
- Shows anxiety
- Has difficulty walking
- Has altered mood

Namaste carers usually first notice signs of discomfort or pain when they are dressing or changing the residents. When the Namaste carer recognizes that pain is present, he or she must immediately notify a nurse who can assess the level or intensity of the pain, the location, and the potential cause. Pain assessment is necessary to determine the appropriate treatment.

Assessment of Pain

Pain can be acute or chronic. Acute pain is usually temporary, such as the pain associated with dental problems or a skin tear. Acute pain will cause the resident to cry out, moan, or have pained facial expressions. This type of pain can be treated with any number of pain medications and usually resolves quickly. The symptoms of a chronic dull pain are more difficult to evaluate and treat. This pain may never totally go away, but it can usually be relieved to the point where it is tolerable.

The first and simplest way to determine if a resident is in pain is to ask. First, touch the resident and get his or her attention, then make eye contact and ask, "Are you in pain?" or "Does anything hurt?" or "Can you show me where it hurts?" If the resident with advanced dementia is not able to understand the meaning of the word *pain* or to communicate the location of the pain, then a pain assessment tool is helpful.

Pain Assessment in Advanced Dementia (PAINAD) is a useful tool for assessing pain in nursing home residents with advanced dementia (see Appendix I). Developed by a team in a dementia unit of a Veterans Hospital, it is adapted from an assessment tool for measuring postoperative pain in young children and is used as a research tool for measuring discomfort. PAINAD is easy to use, objective, reliable, and valid (Warden, Hurley, & Volicer, 2003).

All unresolved pain is reported to the attending physician; if the resident receives the Medicare hospice benefit, hospice nurses are notified. Hospice nurses are specially trained in treating pain and controlling symptoms for individuals who have terminal illnesses. If the pain is unable to be resolved by the attending physician or hospice staff, the services of other professionals may be needed. When the pain originates from the mouth, a dentist may be called to see the resident. If pain is unresolved by routine treatments, other physicians who specialize in pain management may be called for a consultation. Namaste Care nurses should be aggressive in their quest to make residents comfortable.

The resident may have pain from an undiagnosed disease such as cancer. Often, when the resident is in the advanced stage of dementia, testing for cancer is not pursued because of the limited life expectancy of the resident. Surgery is usually not indicated unless it is the only means of keeping the resident comfortable.

Treatment of Pain

When the pain has been assessed for location and intensity, a treatment plan is developed with the physician and documented in the resident's care plan. This most often involves prescribing medications. Pain medications should be given on a regular basis to prevent pain. It takes time for a medication to be effective, and the resident will continue to feel pain for some period of time after the medication is administered. Pain medication should be titrated to a dose that controls pain without producing significant side effects. Breakthrough pain can be treated with a PRN (*pro re nata* or "as needed") order. Giving medications on a regular basis is more beneficial than dispensing medications on a PRN basis.

Residents with advanced dementia sometimes experience difficulties taking oral medication. They may have problems swallowing or spit out the medication, pocket pills in their cheeks, refuse to open their mouths, or chew pills that are not supposed to be chewed. As alternatives, medication may be crushed and given with food, offered in liquid form, inserted rectally, or injected intramuscularly (IM) or subcutaneously (SC).

Intravenous therapy (IV) is a last-resort method of delivering pain medication. In fact, many nursing facilities transfer residents with IV therapy off of the dementia unit to protect them from other well-intentioned residents who try to help by removing the IV. Moving to a new unit, however, takes the resident away from the Namaste team members who know the resident.

If the resident is free from any liver disease, using non-opioid analgesics may be the first treatment choice for mild and moderate chronic pain. Acetaminophen is usually the safest and easiest way to begin treating pain unless the pain is clearly acute. As with any medication, analgesics have benefits and risks that need to be evaluated by the attending physician and side effects that need to be monitored by staff.

When acetaminophen fails to provide relief, the next type of medication that can be ordered is a nonsteroidal anti-inflammatory drug (NSAID) such as ibuprofen. NSAIDs have serious side effects, including gastrointestinal bleeding, so monitoring by all staff is crucial for residents who are taking these medications.

Opiate medications are available to treat pain symptoms that are severe and have not been resolved by non-opioid analgesics or NSAIDs. These drugs, including codeine, fentanyl, and morphine, offer immediate relief. Morphine has fewer side effects than other medications, is effective in relieving severe pain, and can be given in small doses. It can be easily given in liquid form. Morphine is a widely misunderstood drug that many physicians are reluctant to prescribe for residents in nursing homes; nurses are uneasy in administering it; families fear that it will cause their loved one to become overly sedated or addicted to the drug. Some believe that morphine will cause death. Although often given to the resident who is actively dying to ease breathing discomfort, morphine will not cause death when administered in prescribed doses. The most serious side effect is constipation, which can be easily resolved.

The Namaste Care nursing staff needs to become knowledgeable about all aspects of medication types including over-the-counter drugs, usual doses, methods of dispensing, and the conditions under which they are used.

Nontraditional Treatments

Many nontraditional, holistic approaches can enhance well-being and provide comfort. For example, massage therapy can be used to treat pain and discomfort of muscles and joints. The gentle, relaxing strokes may offer comfort to a resident. Reiki is also gaining acceptance from the medical profession. Reiki treatments are being used in hospitals to accelerate healing, relieve pain, lower anxiety, decrease sleep problems, and increase appetites. This technique of laying on hands is used to create life force energy to promote relaxation. Reiki is not a religion and has no harmful effects (Reiki. FAQ, 2006).

Acupuncture is another way of providing relief from pain. This ancient treatment is now being accepted by traditional medicine. Although no research has been done on its use with residents with advanced dementia, it is used to alleviate pain in rehabilitation and acute care settings (Berman et al., 2004).

Aromatherapy and the use of essential oils, especially lavender, geranium, and marjoram, may have calming effects on anxious residents (Flanagan, 1995). These oils should not be used, however, on any resident with allergies. Aromatherapy is a natural, noninvasive treatment system. It has been observed that the aroma of lavender in the Namaste Care room appears to create a calming environment and may be one of the reasons why pacing residents are drawn into the room to sit and rest. Aromatherapy diffusers are available in activity catalogs and are safe to use in the nursing facility environment.

Music is another way to decrease anxiety and lessen pain. Playing soft, tranquil music and nature sounds in a resident's room may help lower anxiety and reduce discomfort. Namaste team members are always exploring ways to help residents feel comfortable. As long as there are no safety concerns and approaches are documented in the care plan, staff should try medical as well as nonmedical holistic approaches to alleviate pain and discomfort.

Monitoring

Once the pain is controlled, regular monitoring, following federal and state guidelines, ensures that the resident is pain free at all times. Some nursing facilities emphasize the importance of monitoring and controlling pain and refer to pain control as the fifth vital sign. James Campbell, M.D., addressed the American Pain Society in 1996, saying, "Vital signs are taken seriously. If pain were assessed with the same zeal as other vital signs, it would have a much better chance of being treated properly. We need to train doctors and nurses to treat pain as a vital sign. Quality care means that pain is measured and treated." The Namaste Care team should constantly monitor pain and discomfort.

ACTIVITIES OF DAILY LIVING

Clothing

Comfort care includes the choice of clothing for residents with advanced dementia. The simplest garments are the best because they make dressing easy. There are companies that specialize in clothing that is easy to use, such as dresses and pants with Velcro fastening. Namaste Care honors the dignity of its residents by making sure they are well dressed and groomed. In the advanced stage of dementia, however, comfort is of primary importance.

Some comfortable options for women include soft sports bras or undershirts instead of traditional bras, slacks with stretchy waistbands, and comfortable blouses and shirts that button or zip in the front. Avoid garments that need to be pulled over the head.

Shoes are not necessary for a resident who is no longer able to ambulate. One facility found it practical to order several dozen slipper socks that were soft and warm and could be easily laundered. With nonskid soles, they are comfortable and safe for those residents who need stability for transferring from a lounge chair to a wheelchair or a bed.

Shorts, even in the summer, may not be appropriate because residents' metabolisms change as they age and older adults tend to be cold. Consider, instead, pants with elastic waistbands and sweatpants.

Educating Namaste team members about how and why residents are dressed is important. The staff should take pride in dressing residents to look their best and may be concerned that a no-shoes policy, for example, would be disrespectful. Staff members may also be concerned that the families might object to comfortable, casual clothing. This becomes less of a concern when the Namaste team members and residents' families are informed that the goal is for residents to feel comfortable in their clothing throughout the day. Families are asked to remove clothing that is not comfortable and to purchase clothing that would be in keeping with the comfort care philosophy. If families disagree with this approach to clothing, their wishes should be respected. Some families insist that shoes are important; others do not like sweatpants. Their requests are always honored. Remember to specify the use of comfortable clothing in the resident's care plan.

Grooming

Comfort approaches should be used in grooming. In addition to washing residents' faces, staff can gently shave faces and brush or comb hair. Safe and appropriate procedures for these activities are described in Chapter 5.

Oral Care

Oral care is very important for residents, and making the procedure comfortable takes sensitivity and special patience from care partners. Residents are usually not able to brush their own teeth and are at risk for oral infections, dental caries, and tarter build-up. The Namaste carer should place a soft toothbrush in a resident's hand in the brushing position to see if the resident remembers how to brush. The Namaste carer might pantomime brushing his or her own teeth as a memory clue. A child's toothbrush may be easier to use than an adult's toothbrush. If a resident is resistive, dipping a mouth swab in something sweet might help induce him or her to submit to some cleaning.

Assessment of the mouth is very important. Namaste carers should notify nurses at once if providing oral care seems to induce pain. Dentists are called if necessary for control of tooth pain. Extracting an infected tooth may be the only way to relieve pain.

Dentures may not be comfortable, particularly for the resident who has lost a great deal of weight. Judge the benefits and comfort of dentures, and discuss this with families. When the residents do not want to wear dentures, they usually find a way to take them out or to communicate their discomfort. Although some families may feel their loved one does not look dignified without teeth, most families agree to discontinue their use if the dentures seem to cause discomfort. Document the decision to remove dentures in the resident's care plan, and be sure to adjust his or her diet accordingly.

Dining and Snacks

Namaste team members make dining a pleasurable experience, even if the resident needs extensive cueing or can no longer feed him- or herself. Residents are encouraged to eat as independently as possible for as long as possible. When they can no longer use utensils, finger foods may help residents to continue feeding themselves for a longer period of time. Cueing with simple instructions, such as, "Mary, please put the spoon in your mouth," and a demonstration of the action can be helpful. Make sure the plate color is different from the food that is placed on it. Consultation with a dietitian may be helpful to identify the best food consistency for each resident.

As dementia progresses, staff must watch residents closely for signs that they are pocketing food, which can lead to choking. If this is the case, physicians usually order special diets containing foods that are easy to swallow. If possible, the staff can ask families what type of comfort food the residents preferred, such as toast, ginger ale, macaroni and cheese, and ice cream.

Assisting residents to eat is a challenge for many nursing facilities when the number of residents needing individual assistance outweighs the number of staff. The regulations in all states prohibit anyone from assisting in the dining room who has not been trained in feeding techniques. Some states mandate that only care partners and nurses can feed residents. Other states require a special training program for anyone feeding residents. Assisting with meals should be a priority for all staff members. Suggestions for how to add extra hands and create a conducive atmosphere at mealtimes include the following:

- Train administrative staff and department managers to assist with dining, if allowed under state regulations.

- Stagger working hours so that extra hands are available in the dining room during the morning and evening meals.

- Hire, train, and pay able seniors to serve as dining assistants.

- Play soft music during meals.

- Make sure dining assistants are talking to the residents, not just among themselves.

- Provide beverages for staff members so that they feel a part of the dining experience.

- Use clothing protectors that do not look like bibs, such as large linen napkins tucked under the chin, bib aprons, or barbecue aprons.

- Discontinue using institutional-looking meal trays.

- If possible, divide residents into small groups to cut down on the noise and confusion of eating in a large room. This can be done inexpensively with large planters or portable privacy screens.

To enhance the experience of dining for residents with advanced dementia, a meeting should be scheduled between Namaste Care team members and the dietitian to brainstorm ways to make the experience of dining a more normal and comforting experience for residents.

Ambulation

Most residents in the advanced stage of dementia are not able to walk, even with assistance. If possible, residents should be evaluated by a physical therapist to ensure that there are no underlying physical reasons for the loss of ambulation. The staff should be trained in the correct approaches to maximize the resident's participation in ambulation or transferring.

When residents in the advanced stage of dementia are not able to safely ambulate, they are confined to a wheelchair. A regular wheelchair may be extremely uncomfortable for residents at this stage of life. The chairs are unbending and do not support the person who cannot sit upright. Each resident in Namaste Care should be assessed to make sure the most comfortable chair is available for them. Wheelchairs or lounge chairs on wheels that can be adjusted are the best choices. Geri-chairs with trays must be assessed to make sure they cannot be viewed as a restraint. Residents enrolled in the Medicare hospice benefit can receive special chairs as part of the durable medical equipment feature. Residents who constantly sit in one place are at great risk of skin breakdown, so care must be taken by Namaste carers to reposition residents at least every 2 hours. Use pillows (consider special lavender-scented pillows) or rolled-up blankets and towels to position residents in their chairs.

Bathing

Of all the personal care procedures, bathing produces the most anxiety in residents with dementia. For them, bathing may be frightening and bewildering. Moving their limbs in the shower or bath can also be painful for residents with joint pain or contractures.

The first step in understanding how to make bathing pleasurable is to find out something about each resident's bathing history. Does she like tub baths, or has she always taken showers? Is he more comfortable and relaxed in the morning, afternoon, or evening? In many instances, the resident has been in the facility for some period of time so the staff knows the resident's preference for bathing. If the resident is new to the facility, families can provide this information. Whoever is making the shower list must understand the resident's preferences and then schedule the appropriate shift for that responsibility. Namaste care partners must also be flexible. If a resident is resistive, staff may approach the resident at a later time or leave bathing for the next shift.

If possible, care partners should take the resident to the bathing area clothed or wearing a bathrobe. If the bathtub is an older model with a lift, hold the resident's hand while he or she is hoisted into the tub. Bathtubs that gradually fill and are easy to enter are the best option. Care partners should have enough towels available to keep the resident covered; if necessary, float a towel on the water to cover the resident or have the person wear a hospital gown.

Following facility bathing procedures, Namaste carers should talk to residents throughout the bathing sequence. In a soothing voice, they should tell the resident what they are doing, ask the resident to hold the soap (if he or she will not eat it) or the washcloth, and make the resident feel that he or she is participating. Another approach is to talk about everything but the bath to distract the resident from the bathing experience.

Showers might be less traumatic with one of the new large shower heads that create the feeling of being in a gentle rain. Hand-held shower heads are also good to use, as the resident has some control over the direction of the spray. Playing music during the bath or shower and making sure the room is warm help to reduce anxiety and increase the comfort of bathing. Battery-powered radios are safer than electrical appliances in the bathing area. Also consider warming a blanket in a microwave oven to wrap around the resident after bathing. After the bath, staff should apply lotion to the resident's body and give a back rub. With a bit of ingenuity, bathing even the most resistive resident is possible.

SAM

Sam was impossible to bathe. He did not recognize his wife of many years, and he sure did not want this stranger to assist him in the tub or shower. She was at her wits end until she realized that her husband was a very sound sleeper and she could wash about a third of his body before he woke up. Giving a complete bed bath took some time, but eventually he was completely washed!

Bed Baths

Bed baths are often the preferred bathing method for residents in Namaste Care who are resistive to tub baths or showers, are ill, have extreme joint pain, or are actively dying. Bed baths are comfortable and are given in the privacy of the resident's room. Bed bath techniques may need to be reviewed with nursing assistants.

The staff on a dementia unit at the Bedford, Massachusetts, Veteran's Hospital decided to study whether reminiscence during bathing would lower resistance. Nurses were hired for the study and trained in using reminiscence as an intervention. Care partners and nurses on the dementia unit selected the most resistant residents for the study. The nurses decided to do bed baths with the reminiscence; when they used this method of bathing even without reminiscence, the resistiveness to bathing disappeared (Mahoney et al., 1999), demonstrating that bed baths are less upsetting.

To give a bed bath, first gather all necessary supplies; this includes soap, two basins of warm water (one for washing and one for rinsing), face cloths, towels, lotion, and dry shampoo. Clean clothing and personal grooming items such as moisturizer, combs, and brushes are also good to have available. Playing music and making sure the room is warm help to make the environment cozy and the experience soothing. Remember, bathing has the potential of being a pleasant experience; it just takes a bit of ingenuity.

Comforting Environment

Little research has been done on how and if the environment of nursing facility residents with advanced dementia provides comfort (Calkins, 2003). Namaste Care is built on honoring the person in every way possible, so providing an attractive and comforting environment is important. Chapter 6 provides many ideas on how to make the Namaste Care room and a Namaste Care wing look warm and inviting.

The residents' rooms, where they spend many hours, should also be as comfortable as possible. Rooms should be personalized with pictures and other familiar items; be sure to place these items where residents can see them. One enterprising facility painted the ceilings in residents' rooms with clouds and birds. Another facility repainted each room as they had funds available. Another facility asked organizations and private benefactors to adopt a resident's room. Some of the donations were monetary and some took the form of volunteers to paint the rooms.

SUMMARY

Namaste Care recognizes that in order to provide a quality of life for residents, eliminating pain and discomfort must be a top priority. Comfort care must include both medical interventions, such as pain and symptom management, and the more psychosocial aspects of care. Psychosocial aspects include the way residents are bathed and assisted with activities of daily living, how they are dressed and seated in chairs, and how meaningful their activities are made.

One family member commented, "I feel as if I am enveloped in a cocoon of comfort and love," to express how she felt when she walked onto the Namaste Care wing. Namaste Care honored not only her husband, but also her as part of the Namaste Care family. Comfort care provides a lifestyle that lessens the tragedy of dementia. When residents are comfortable, the staff feels better too. When residents are comfortable, families feel better about visiting their loved ones and less anxious when they leave them.

Matthew's Story

Matthew's comfort was very important to his wife Celia. She visited several times a week and said it was so much easier to leave him when he was comfortable and in no apparent distress. His half of the room was decorated with pictures of their five children and numerous grandchildren. Celia also bought a quilt for his bed.

Showers had always been Matthew's preferred method of bathing, and staff usually had no trouble bathing him when they showed him Celia's picture and reminded him he had a date with her. As Matthew became less and less verbal, his Namaste carers learned to read his nonverbal communication and kept him comfortable. He never appeared to be in pain, but staff members constantly monitored him. Matthew was dressed in clothing that was comfortable and warm. His family was reassured that he was at ease in his surroundings, which comforted his wife and children as they faced the loss of their beloved husband and father. They knew that Dad was in the capable hands of the Namaste Care team.

CHAPTER 9

Dying and Death

When a resident begins to actively die, Namaste team members are prepared to help the resident make the transition from life to death in a peaceful, dignified manner and, whenever possible, in the presence of others. It is up to the living to help write the final chapter of the residents' lives. For the families, this leave-taking will remain in their mind's eye forever, and the Namaste Care team will do everything possible to make this memory serene.

Years ago, care of the sick and dying was the duty of families. Death took place at home with relatives, who were also the primary caregivers. Family members may have even prepared the body after death. People knew and understood that this was one of their roles and responsibilities; just as they assisted with the birthing of new babies, they also cared for the dying. Now, however, in spite of the wonderful work of hospice, many people with a terminal illness die in a hospital or in a nursing facility (Mitchell, Teno, Miller, & Mor, 2005). There are more than 3,000 hospice programs operating in the United States serving more than 900,000 patients annually (Connor, Tecca, Lund, Person, & Teno, 2004).

Namaste Care encourages death to occur in the resident's home, the nursing facility. Transferring the resident who is actively dying to a hospital will not change the outcome. In fact, the trauma of moving the resident to a hospital may hasten the death. The nursing home is

the resident's home, and the staff has become family—a family that is
skilled at providing palliative care for a dying resident.

SIGNS OF IMPENDING DEATH

One of the first signs that a resident is entering the last days of life
may be an unresponsiveness to activities in the Namaste Care room.
In addition, the resident will sleep most of the time and will be difficult to arouse. He or she may not be able to open or focus the eyes
when spoken to and be uninterested in food and beverages; even the
beloved lollipops are no longer tempting. At the approach of these
signs, Namaste carers shift their focus to providing care for the
dying resident and grief support for the family.

During this time, it is beneficial for the resident to be in a quiet,
comfortable place, away from the Namaste Care room. When residents live in a shared room, closing the privacy curtains will offer
some seclusion. Whenever possible, remove the roommate to the
Namaste Care room, an activity area, or some other common space.
This will provide some privacy for the family and the dying resident.
Nursing facilities that offer Namaste Care are encouraged to designate a private room that can be reserved for residents who are actively dying, such as the Reagan Room discussed in Chapter 6.

The Namaste Care commitment continues to honor the spirit
within as the resident begins to actively die. The resident may appear quiet and tranquil. The focus is on making the resident as
comfortable as possible. It is important that those who remain, staff
as well as family members, be honorable witnesses to this last miracle of life and take away good memories of this death.

Nurses are usually the first to recognize when a resident is actively dying. They are often alerted by a care partner who has observed a significant decline in the resident's physical status or has an
inner sense that the dying process has begun. When residents cross
the threshold and begin to actively die, they may experience a significant decrease in their functional states. For example, they are

- Unable to turn in bed without assistance
- Incontinent of urine and unable to control bowel function
- Difficult or impossible to arouse

- Not hungry; eating or drinking very little or not at all
- Unable to focus their eyes; eyes may have a glazed appearance

In most cases, residents with advanced dementia give signals when they are actively dying. Sally Smith (1998), a nurse practitioner working with residents in a nursing facility, has written about the dying process and identified what happens to the body in this last stage of life. She also provided ideas on how staff and families can care for nursing facility residents as they are dying. Namaste team members should be aware of these signs and be able to show families how they can still help to provide loving care.

Decreased Appetite

When the body begins the process of shutting down, the need or desire for food diminishes significantly. It is believed that this is the body's way of protecting itself. Without food, there is no danger of choking or vomiting during the dying process. When the resident stops eating, endorphins are released that reduce pain. Feeding tubes and hydration block the release of endorphins and can lead to discomfort. For several days or hours prior to the actual death, the resident often refuses all offers of food or beverage. Withdrawing from food and liquid is just part of the natural process of the body preparing for death.

During this time, the resident's lips and mouth might look parched. Care partners and the resident's family can help moisturize the mouth area by using swabs that contain lemon glycerin or another moisturizing agent. Ice chips placed below the tongue or in the cheek and artificial saliva may also be used to provide moisture in the mouth. Small spoonfuls of soft ice cream may still be enjoyed by the resident and will help moisten the lips and tongue. Care partners and family members should watch the resident's facial expressions to assess if any of these options are uncomfortable for the resident.

Family and Namaste team members believe that they should be doing something and often feel helpless. Doing, however, is less important to the dying person than it is for us, the care partners. Bill Thomas, the physician who began the Eden Alternative, expresses his feelings about what many perceive as doing nothing. He speaks of the difference between doing and being and how hard it is for most of us just to *be*. For those of us observing the dying process, we can *be* beside the person. We can *be* present with all of our energy (W. Thomas, personal communication). And that is, very simply, enough.

Lethargy

As dementia progresses, the resident becomes more and more lethargic, sleeping for longer periods of time. When the resident reaches the actively dying stage, it will become difficult, if not impossible, to arouse him or her. This person will sleep most of the time. Namaste carers and family members can read to the dying resident, play music the resident enjoyed in the past, and just be present.

Skin Changes

As the body begins to cease functioning, the heart rate may become rapid or may decrease significantly. The surface of the skin becomes cool and moist. Color begins to disappear until the skin appears almost transparent. The circulation of blood in the body is slowing, impairing the flow to hands and feet. The hands, nail beds, and feet begin to get cyanotic, turning a bluish hue or looking mottled or blotchy. These are natural signs of impending death that can be frightening for the family. Tuck soft, warm blankets or sheets around the resident for comfort if he or she appears cold. Keep warm socks on the resident's feet, and gently rub warm lotion or baby oil onto the skin.

Fever

Occasionally, the actively dying resident will have a fever. This may be due to dehydration or an infection. Fever can be controlled with medication if it appears that the resident is uncomfortable. The resident needs to be observed closely to monitor pain and discomfort. It is difficult to administer medication when the person is in the actively dying state; however, medication may be given rectally or in liquid form if the resident can still swallow. The best treatment may be applying a cool facecloth on the face and limbs. If a fever is present, Namaste carers should watch for it to break, as the bed linens will need to be changed at that time.

Kidney Function

As the resident's body is shutting down, the kidneys begin to cease normal functioning, and the body simply does not make very much urine. The resident has no bladder or bowel control, so he or she may be constantly leaking urine and feces. Even a small amount of urine or feces will make the skin tender, so it is necessary to check the skin on a frequent basis to make sure it is clean and lubricated. There is no need for a catheter at this point.

Breathing

The respiratory system begins to shut down as the resident approaches the final hours of life. Breathing may become labored. Most people with Alzheimer's disease (AD) die from pneumonia. Although the process may not be painful for the resident, it is very painful for the family to watch. Morphine in low doses eases the breathing and will not hasten death. Oxygen administered by a nasal cannula can also ease breathing. Other medications can be administered if the resident seems anxious or distressed during the dying process.

Loose secretions in the chest are another symptom of impending death. These are not painful to the resident, but the rasping or rattling it adds to breathing can be upsetting for families to hear. Placing the resident on his or her side may help the fluid drain naturally. In fact, the natural dehydration that occurs is actually helpful in preventing fluid buildup. Avoid suctioning; it is uncomfortable, does not have any lasting benefit for the resident, and is not part of the Namaste Care approach. Remember that families will need constant reassurance that their loved one is not suffering, even though it sounds as if the resident is experiencing discomfort.

In the last few hours or minutes of life, breathing is very irregular. This can seem like an agonizing end to a difficult journey for the family. It may be helpful to the family to have someone else present at this time. Because families may need to feel useful, encourage members to read from a Bible or other religious or spiritual book or to hold their loved one's hands. Namaste team members should constantly reassure families of the importance of being physically close to their loved ones. Holding hands is a loving connection. Sometimes family members will want to lie next to their loved ones, a caring touch that easily communicates love when words fail.

When the signs of impending death appear, families may become frightened. They become alarmed when they see the changes in the body and do not understand that what they are observing is the natural process of death. Namaste care partners should help families understand the physical changes and assure them that the process of dying is not painful.

NAMASTE CARE PROTOCOL
FOR ACTIVELY DYING RESIDENTS

When the Namaste Care nursing staff recognizes that a resident is actively dying, they may follow a protocol:

- The nurse in charge of the unit calls the resident's physician to inform him or her of the status of the patient and ask for comfort care orders. These may include orders not to hospitalize and not to resuscitate as well as orders for oxygen to assist breathing and morphine or other medications to ease discomfort.

- The family is notified of the resident's declining condition by the charge nurse or social worker. If the facility has a private room available, such as the Reagan Room, the family is asked if it would like to move the resident to this room. A Namaste team member should explain that if the resident recovers from this episode, he or she will be returned to his or her original room.

- When the resident is receiving hospice care, the hospice nurse is summoned and involved in calling the physician and the family. The hospice staff and Namaste Care nursing staff work as a team so that families are not confused by differing opinions and information.

- When the Reagan Room is used, housekeeping is notified to make sure the room is readied for the resident's arrival. Prior to moving the resident, soft music is played to welcome the resident and personal pictures from the resident's room are brought into the room. Often, a plant or flowers can be borrowed from somewhere in the building.

- The medical equipment needed to make the resident more comfortable needs to be brought into the room. Oxygen and personal supplies such as mouth swabs, face cloths, towels, and basins are stocked.

- If the resident is transferred to another room, the business office and nursing department must be notified. Regulations state that the resident's name must be posted outside his or her room. Bookkeeping records must also be kept current.

- The family is asked if anyone else should be contacted, such as a close friend or clergy member.

- If a priest, minister, or rabbi is in the facility, he or she is notified that a resident is dying and is asked to stop by to offer consolation to family members. The family may wish to have a special clergy member contacted, which would usually be handled by the facility social worker. If the resident is receiving hospice services, the hospice clergy person may be notified by the hospice nurse.

- The dietary department is notified so that soft ice cream, juices, ice chips, and other beverages can be made available for the resident. The dietary department also provides beverages and meals for the family and visitors.

- Social work staff members are notified so that they can make themselves available for family members of the dying resident.

Each facility providing Namaste Care should develop its own protocol. This protocol becomes a valuable tool, especially when the charge nurse is new or not familiar with the procedures of the facility.

IN THE PRESENCE OF OTHERS

David Kessler (1997) wrote about "walking people to the gate." Prior to September 11th, 2001, travelers were walked to the gate at the train station, bus station, or airport. They could wave good-bye and give a parting hug or kiss to their loved ones. This concept of caring for the dying, in fact walking them to the gate, is a good way to visualize staying by the side of a dying person until he or she leaves us. The Namaste Care team makes every effort to ensure that residents do not die alone.

Some families want to know when the end is near so that they can be with their loved ones; others cannot bear to see the person die. Some residents have outlived their family members, or families are not able to get to the facility before the resident dies. Many studies have revealed that elderly people do not fear death but do not want to die alone or in pain (MetLife Foundation, 2006). When the Namaste Care team recognizes the signs of impending death and no family is available, arrangements should be made for someone to be present with the resident. Following are some ideas for recruiting volunteers to sit by the side of a dying resident:

- Ask department managers to take work, such as charting, to the bedside. Residents at this point do not need conversation, just someone to sit with them and occasionally touch them.

- See if the resident's church has volunteers who can spend time with the resident.

- Develop a relationship with a hospice program that will offer volunteers to be present for the dying, even if the resident is not a hospice patient.

- Provide special training to senior volunteers who are willing to sit with dying residents.

- Schedule a care partner who is on light or limited duty to sit in the room.

- Ask all staff members in the facility to sign up for 30-minute intervals.

The following example of a resident with no close family shows the commitment of the Namaste Care team:

MAY

> May had never married and had outlived most of her family and friends. She had one nephew who visited her occasionally but otherwise was alone. May had been on the Namaste Care wing for about 6 months when one of the care partners told me that she thought May was dying. When asked why she thought that, she shrugged and said it was just a sense she had that May was getting ready to leave us. A few weeks later, on my next visit to the facility, May was in the Reagan Room. Her pictures were hung on the wall, a rosary was in her hand, and a care partner was sitting with her.
>
> Her nephew had been called, but he was unable to come, so the staff stepped in and became her family. One care partner came in on her day off just to be with May. It was moving to see this resident, who had almost no family and no friends, die peacefully holding the hand of someone who cared and wept as May died.

David Kessler (1997) stated, "Death by nature is one of the most isolating experiences we can ever have." Families who want someone to be with the dying person every moment may have unrealistic expectations. Namaste Care team members should explain to families about the timing of death. From my experience and reading on the subject, *when* people choose to leave is a very personal decision. Families feel so much guilt when they leave the room for a few minutes or go home for something and the person dies. But some people cannot die with family members in the room. The following story is an example:

JANE

> Jane was dying of cancer. Her husband Robert, their six children, and Robert's mother were in the hospital room watching over Jane after having been told she would not live through the day. It was a Catholic hospital and when Mass was announced over the loudspeaker, Robert asked the kids to go and pray for their mother. As soon as they left the room, Jane took her last breath. She apparently could not die in the presence of her children.

My own parents taught me about choosing the time to die. My father evidently wanted me, his only child, to be with him at the end. Daddy was in a coma for many hours. Eventually, I needed to get some sleep and went home. As an only child, it was up to me to make all of the funeral arrangements. The hospital staff agreed to call me when he died. The next morning when I woke up, I realized the hospital had not called. I phoned the nurse's station and was told that he was still alive. I raced to the hospital, entered his hospital room, and lay next to him. I said, "Daddy, you waited," and he took his last breath. My mother, on the other hand, lingered until my father left the hospital before she died. I think she knew he did not want to see her die. Even with the knowledge we have about the last stages of life and the dying process, most experts agree that dying is as individual as each person's life experience.

If possible, someone should be with the family at the time of death, prepared for whatever emotions are expressed and ready to offer support. When my mother died, a nurse stayed with me, standing quietly behind me as I said my final good-bye. It was a good thing he did because my mother's body began to move and, thinking she was still alive, I panicked. The nurse gently touched my shoulder, explaining that this was a normal reaction after death.

The Namaste Care team members must also monitor the reactions of family members as the dying process comes to an end. Tissues, some beverages, and a handy chair should be available for family members who look as if they might faint. Families, and even individual family members, differ in their comfort levels with the dying process. Some family members cannot touch the person as they are dying. In this case, the Namaste care partner can hold the family member's hand and the dying resident's hand, connecting all in a circle of love. Others want to be as close as possible. The double bed in the Reagan Room is a wonderful asset to the family member who wants to lie next to his or her loved one. Namaste Care team members are nonjudgmental about the actions and reactions of families during this time. Just as they are present for the person who is dying, they must also be present for that person's family.

Matthew's Story

As a consultant, I am rarely with residents at the end of life, so it was an honor for me to be visiting on July 12 and to witness Matthew's death. When the Namaste carer who had been staying with the couple was needed to help feed other residents, I stayed with Celia. We both held Matthew's hands and did our best to help him to the end of this voyage. Although not a nurse, I have been present at enough deaths to explain what was happening to his body. Celia became upset when Matthew's hands began to turn blue and his breathing became irregular. I suggested that she cover him with another blanket and hold his hand. Celia's face glowed as she held her husband's hand and told stories of their life together and of the special family they had raised. It was a beautiful sight, tears streaming down her face and love shining through her eyes. Matthew was a very fortunate man to have Celia beside him, literally "till death do us part."

Celia talked to Matthew as if he could hear her. She told him how much she loved him and how she cherished the years they had together. She told him she was fine and that, although she would miss him, she would be all right; he could leave with her love. Jennie, the charge nurse, walked in the room and realized that death was imminent, so she stayed at our side. Both Jennie and I were crying. How wonderful, I thought, that after seeing so many deaths we could still cry when a resident died.

Matthew would take a breath and then stop, and we would all think he had left us; then he would take another breath. This seemed to go on for a long time. Something seemed to be holding Matthew back. Then Celia told a comical story about their life together; we all laughed, and off he went on the wings of laughter. We hugged Celia and she said her final good-bye to her dear husband, Matthew.

Death is always sad, perhaps heartbreaking, but a good death can be filled with reassuring memories of the last moments of life, with the gentleness and serenity with which a loved one slipped away in harmony with the world.

FAMILIES' REACTIONS TO THE DEATH

Some families want to stay in the room with the body for awhile; others leave immediately. Making sure that the family's wishes are honored at this time is important. Death can be pronounced by either a nurse or a physician, depending on the state in which the facility is located. Families may need time to adjust to the actual death before a nurse or physician actually pronounces it. When family members are ready, they will be asked to leave the room while the body is prepared for the funeral home personnel. For the family and staff this is a time of conflicting feelings; both sadness and a sense of relief are tangled together. Most families have lived with the disease for so many years that the finality of death, while devastating, finally brings an end to the unrelenting assault of AD.

Namaste Care is about care for the families as well as for the residents. Staff now is caring for the family, making sure the family members are not alone after they leave the facility. Many of the surviving spouses are elderly and may have health problems, so find out if they have someone to be with them before they leave the facility. The staff should evaluate the safety of the spouse if he or she is driving home alone. At this time, having a friend or clergy member present help puts everyone at ease. When no one is available, someone from the facility should take the spouse home and stay until he or she is able to be alone.

Families may be in shock after the death and not be able to remember things such as contacting their children, friends, or clergy. It is a very good idea for the social worker to make sure that all pertinent information is easily located in the resident's chart so that someone can assist the family in making these calls.

Some families are relieved after the death. They are exhausted from being observers as this cruel disease claimed the person they loved, bit by bit. How families react is very individual; Namaste Care team members should consider themselves to be shepherds guiding families along the end of the journey and ensuring their safety. Namaste Care continues after the resident has died.

AFTER-DEATH CARE

Autopsy

Some families decide to have an autopsy. Autopsy literally means to *see for yourself*. It is a special surgical operation performed by a physician. It is done in a respectful manner in a laboratory or in a funeral home. Signs often posted in autopsy laboratories say, "This is the place where death rejoices to teach those who live."

The decision about having an autopsy must be made prior to death or directly after the death, depending on state regulations. The reasons why people choose to have an autopsy are varied. Some families need to know if their loved one really had AD, a definitive diagnosis that can only be reached after the brain has been examined by an autopsy. Diagnostic criteria are so advanced now that brains that have been studied after death show that 90% of the diagnoses of "probable" AD are accurate. To be 100% accurate, an autopsy must take place. Results are available within 3 months.

Some residents have been enrolled in research programs that have an autopsy as part of their protocol. In those cases, the facility should have the information about who to inform when the resident has died so that the autopsy can be done within the appropriate time frame.

One of the greatest fears of families considering autopsy is that the body will be disfigured. This is not true. An incision is made in the back of the scalp and the scar is not visible. Most religions allow this procedure. If the family is in doubt, their religious or spiritual adviser can assist in making the decision.

Brain and Organ Donation

Donating a brain or any part of the body to research may be some residents' final gift. If someone does choose to donate a part of his or her body to research, the Namaste Care team members should be informed by the family to ensure that the person's wishes are carried out. The Alzheimer's Association has information regarding brain autopsy, and many research centers also have literature regarding donations. The medical record should contain information on the resident's wish to make an organ donation as well as instructions on disposition of the body.

Preparation of the Body

The Namaste Care nursing staff prepares the body for the funeral home following the facility nursing procedures. If the family was not with the resident when he or she died, the nurse needs to call and inform them about the death. Family members are asked if they wish to see the body before the funeral home is called. Sometimes, they are on their way to the facility when the resident dies. In these cases, the Namaste Care team prepares the room and the resident so that everything looks as peaceful as possible.

The resident is cleaned and dressed in fresh pajamas or a nightgown, not a hospital gown. Hair is combed and neatly groomed. After a person dies, the skin takes on a grayish hue; the face is devoid of color. A bit of light lipstick for the ladies and a touch of rouge can improve the appearance of the skin. All medical equipment is taken from the room. Music is playing and lights are dimmed. An over-the-bed table containing the resident's personal pictures and flowers is a nice touch.

When the family arrives, someone from the Namaste Care team who feels particularly close to the family, or the person who was with the resident as he or she died, walks into the room with the family. Tissues should be available. Family members are asked if they want someone to stay in the room with them or if they want to be alone. Some families need someone to be with them. Others just need to be alone. If families wish to be left alone, have a Namaste Care team member check in periodically.

Taking the Resident Out of the Facility

Years ago, residents' bodies were hidden from other residents as the gurney was being wheeled out of the facility. When a death occurred, residents were taken to their rooms and all of the doors were shut. The body would be quickly wheeled through the corridor and then staff would let everyone out of their rooms. Of course, the first question out of the residents' mouths was, "Who died?"

The subject of death, while not completely out of the shadows, is taking steps toward the light of reality. Death is not a fearful subject for the residents, and honoring residents' bodies as they leave the facility is not upsetting for residents. The Namaste Care ritual honors residents even after death has occurred and they are leaving the facility.

When the body is ready to leave the room, Namaste Care team members place a quilt or flag over it. The gurney is wheeled out, accompanied by family, friends, and staff. Sometimes a prayer is read as the gurney is being placed in the hearse. Most of the time, the team member walking beside the gurney places his or her hand on the body, reassuring the resident that even in death he or she is not alone.

Matthew's Story

After Matthew died, Celia requested some time alone with her husband. When she was ready to leave the room, Namaste Care team members came in to clean and dress Matthew. All medical equipment was taken from the room and the bedside table was arranged with his pictures, a live plant, and a small flag to pay homage to his years of service in the military. Celia then sat with him until the funeral home attendants arrived. She left the room while his body was put on the gurney. An American flag was placed over Matthew and, with his wife Celia, the charge nurse, a care partner, and other staff, he left the place that had been his home for several years. As they walked alongside the gurney, everyone touched Matthew. When they reached the hearse, the gurney was placed in the back, and the Namaste carer read a brief poem. Then, at this very sad moment when the hearse was leaving, everyone spontaneously waved; realizing what they had done, they laughed and cried and hugged each other as Matthew was slowly driven away.

Celia later remarked that the experience of her husband's death was beautiful, even peaceful. She was so surprised that, although sad, she felt honored that staff was with her and shared the final moments. Accompanying Matthew to the hearse provided her with a sense of closure, and she had an overwhelming feeling of peace. She said, "I'm glad I stayed to the end. I would not have wanted to miss this last part of our journey together."

After the deceased resident is taken from the building, Namaste Care continues. The bed is stripped and remade with a bedspread and pillow. Namaste Care team members often talk about how sad they feel if the bed is left unmade after a resident they have cared for dies; there is nothing to show that a person lived and died in that room. Instead, care partners make the bed with just a bedspread (because fresh linen will be needed when a new resident is admitted) and place a silk rose on the bed along with a picture or some other personal item of the resident. Usually, management allows this memorial to stay on the bed for at least 24 hours. This seems to help the staff to grieve; it gives everyone time to adjust to the death before another resident is moved to the bed.

Clothing and other personal items are packed in boxes, never garbage bags, and stored in a safe place until the family is available to pick them up or indicates that they should be donated to other residents.

TAKING CARE OF THE NAMASTE CARE TEAM

After the resident has left the building, someone needs to thank the Namaste Care team members for the loving care they have given to the resident. The charge nurse usually gathers the facility staff for this acknowledgment and also informs the incoming staff members of the death, thanking them for their care as well. It is helpful for the Namaste Care team members, many of whom feel like they have lost a friend or relative, to hear the positive details surrounding the death, such as that the resident died peacefully and was surrounded by family. All staff members, even though they deal with death more than the average person, still need reassurance that the death was a good death and that they made a difference in the quality of life and death of the resident.

We must never forget how much the staff cares about the residents. Many staff members need to talk about favorite residents long after a death has occurred. One resident who paced all day unless he was coaxed into the Namaste Care room is always remembered when the Namaste carers look at "his" couch. His spirit remains in the thoughts of staff, as do the spirits of so many residents who have lived and died in nursing facilities.

Bereavement Services

Within a day after the death, the social worker should circulate a sympathy card on the unit and ask all Namaste Care team members to sign it. Department managers and the administrator should also sign it. Make sure that someone from the facility can attend the funeral or the viewing; it is a gesture that means so much to the family and is helpful to the grieving staff.

Evaluation of Care

Several days after the death, a brief meeting needs to be held for each shift that helped care for the deceased resident. The purpose is to evaluate the effectiveness of Namaste Care. Facilitated by the social worker or charge nurse, the Namaste Care team is asked questions related to the resident's time in Namaste Care and whether the resident's death was

- Pain free
- Peaceful
- Without signs of distress
- With family present and supported

At the end of the meeting, the resident is honored with a brief period of silence; then, memories of the resident are shared. These usually produce laughter and the meeting ends, much like our friend Matthew's life did, with joy.

Matthew's Story

After Matthew's death, the grieving process began with small reminders to staff that Matthew Wilk had lived and died in the Reagan Room. Namaste Care team members were thanked by the family and by department managers for their part in helping to make Matthew's death a "good death." A memorial service was held later in the week.

It is my fervent wish that everyone living with dementia could experience the equivalent of Matthew's "good death." Without seeing it firsthand, it is impossible to imagine the magic created within the

Namaste Care room and through the special care provided by Namaste carers. I have had the privilege of implementing numerous Namaste Care programs and in every one staff members have been amazed by the peace that falls over the residents in Namaste Care. I hope, therefore, that you will put your arms around Namaste Care and advocate for your residents who have advanced dementia. Thank you for taking time to read this book.

Namaste!

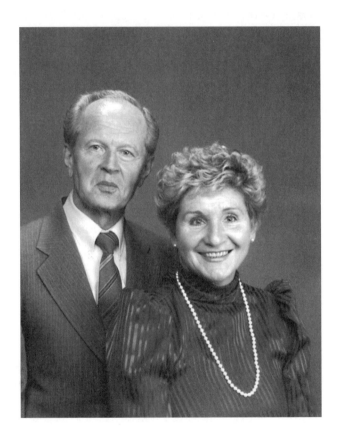

References

Alzheimer's Association. (2005). *Dementia care practice recommendations for assisted living residences and nursing homes.* Chicago: Alzheimer's Association.

Alzheimer's Association. (2006). Retrieved on line at www.alz.org/maintain yourbrain/overview.asp

Alzheimer's Association. (2007). Retrieved May 15, 2007 on line at www.alz.org/about_us_about_us.asp

Bell, V., & Troxel, D. (1996, 2003). *The Best Friends approach to Alzheimer's care.* Baltimore: Health Professions Press.

Berman, B.M., Lao, L., Langenberg, P., et al. (2004). Effectiveness of acupuncture as adjunctive therapy in osteoarthritis of the knee: A randomized controlled trial. *Annals of Internal Medicine, 141,* 901–910.

Brawley, E.C. (1997). *Designing for Alzheimer's disease: Strategies for creating better care environments.* New York: John Wiley & Sons, Inc.

Brawley, E.C. (2006). *Designing innovations for aging and Alzheimer's.* New York: John Wiley & Sons, Inc.

Calkins, M. (2003). Research impacting design impacting research. *Alzheimer's Care Quarterly, 4,* 172–176.

Calkins, M. (2005). Environments for late-stage dementia. *Alzheimer's Care Quarterly, 6,* 71–75.

Callahan, S. (2005). Spiritual connections. *Alzheimer's Care Quarterly, 6,* 4–13.

Camberg, L., Woods, P., Ooi, W.L., Hurley, A., Volicer, L., Ashley, J., et al. (1999). Evaluation of Simulated Presence: A personalized approach to enhance well-being in persons with Alzheimer's disease. *Journal of the American Geriatrics Society, 47,* 446–452.

Centers for Medicare and Medicaid Services (CMS). (2002). Available on line at www.cms.hhs.gov/NursingHomeQualityInits.

Connor, S.R., Tecca, M., Lund, Person, J., & Teno, J. (2004). Measuring hospice care: The National Hospice and Palliative Care Organization National Hospice Data Set. *Journal of Pain Symptom Management, 28,* 316–328.

Cuddy, L.L., & Duffin, J. (2005). Music, memory, and Alzheimer's disease: Is music recognition spared in dementia, and how can it be assessed? *Medical Hypotheses, 64,* 229–235.

Decker, F.H., Gruhn, P., Matthews-Martin, L., & et al. (2006). 2002 AHCA survey of nursing staff vacancy and turnover in nursing homes. Retrieved on line at www.ahca/research/rpt_vts2002_final.pfd

Evans, D.A., Funkenstein, H.H., Albert, M.S., Scherr, P.A., Cook, N.R., Chown, M.J., et al. (1989). Prevalence of Alzheimer's disease in a community population of older persons: Higher than previously reported. *Journal of the American Medical Association, 262,* 2551–2556.

Feil, N. (1982). *V/F Validation: The Feil method.* Cleveland: Edward Feil Productions.

Feil, N. (2002). *The validation breakthrough* (2nd ed.). Baltimore: Health Professions Press.

Finucane, T.E., Christmas, C., & Travis, K. (1999). Tube feeding in patients with advanced dementia: A review of the evidence. *Journal of the American Medical Association, 282,* 1365–1370.

Flanagan, N. (1995). Essential oils and aromatherapy for Alzheimer's patients. *Alternative & Complementary Therapies,* 377–380.

Fried, T.R., Gillick, M.R., & Lipsitz, L.A. (1995). Whether to transfer? Factors associated with hospitalization and outcome of elderly long-term care patients with pneumonia. *Journal of General Internal Medicine, 10,* 246–250.

Ghusan, H.F., Teasdale, T.A., Pepe, P.E., & Ginger, V.F. (1995). Older nursing home residents have a cardiac arrest survival rate similar to that of older persons living in the community. *Journal of the American Geriatrics Society, 43,* 520–527.

Gillick, M.R., & Mitchell, S.L. (2002). Facing eating difficulties in end-stage dementia. *Alzheimer's Care Quarterly, 3,* 227–232.

Hellen, C.R. (1997). Communications and fundamentals of care: Bathing, grooming, and dressing. In C.R. Kovach (Ed.), *Late-stage dementia care: A basic guide* (pp. 113–125). Washington, DC: Taylor & Francis.

Huffman, J.C., & Kunik, M.E. (2000). Assessment and understanding of pain in patients with dementia. *Gerontologist, 40,* 574–581.

Kessler, D. (1997). *The rights of the dying.* New York: HarperCollins.

Kitwood, T. (1998). Toward a theory of dementia care: Ethics and interaction. *Journal of Clinical Ethics, 9,* 23–34.

Kübler-Ross, E. (1969). On death and dying. New York: Macmillan.

Mahoney et al. (1999). Reducing uncomfortable behaviors when bathing persons with Alzheimer's disease: What kind of evidence for choosing interventions? *Neurobiological Aging, 23,* S92.

Maurer, K., Volk, S., & Gerbaldo, H. (1997). Auguste D and Alzheimer's disease. *Lancet, 349,* 1546–1549.

Maust, D.T., Onyike, C.U., Sheppard, J.M., Mayer, L.S., Samus, Q.M., et al. (2006). Predictors of caregiver unawareness and nontreatment of dementia among residents of assisted living facilities: The Maryland assisted living study. *American Journal of Geriatric Psychiatry, 14,* 668–675.

MetLife Foundation. (2006). Americans fear Alzheimer's more than heart disease, diabetes or stroke, but few prepare. Retrieved on line at www.metlife.com/applications/Corporate/wps/cda/pagegenerator/0,4132,P12046,00.html

Miller, L., & Talerico, K.A. (2005). Development of an intervention to reduce pain in older adults with dementia. *Alzheimer's Care Quarterly, 6,* 154–167.

Mitchell, S.L., Teno, J.M., Miller, S.C., & Mor, V. (2005). A national study of the location of death for older persons with dementia. *Journal of the American Geriatrics Society, 53,* 299–305.

Morrison, R.S., Ahronheim, J.C., Morrison, G.R., Darling, E., Baskin, S.A., Morris, J., et al. (1998). Pain and discomfort associated with common hospital procedures and experiences. *Journal of Pain & Symptom Management, 15,* 91–101.

National Center for Health Statistics. (2006). National Home and Hospice Care data. Retrieved on line at www.cdc.gov/nchs/about/major/nhhcsd/nhhschomecare3.htm

Orr-Rainey, N. (1994). The evolution of special care units: The nursing home industry perspective. *Journal of Alzheimer's Disease and Associated Disorders, 8,* 139–143.

Orsulic-Jeras, S., Judge, K.S., & Camp, C.J. (2000). Montessori-based activities for long-term care residents with advanced dementia: Effects on engagement and affect. *Gerontologist, 40,* 107–111.

Patient Self-Determination Act, P.L. 101-508, 42 U.S.C.§ 1395 & 4751.

Pioneer Network. (2006). Retrieved on line at www.pioneernetwork.net.

Reiki FAQ. (2006). Retrieved on line at www.reiki.org/FAQ/WhatIsReiki.html

Simard, J. (2000). The Memory Enhancement Program: A new approach to increasing the quality of life for people with mild memory loss. In S.M. Albert (Ed.), *Assessing quality of life in Alzheimer's disease* (pp. 153–162). New York: Springer Publishing.

Simard, J. (2005). Namaste: Giving life to the end of life. *Alzheimer's Care Quarterly, 6,* 14–19.

Simard, J., & Volicer, L. (2002). The Club: Increasing the quality of life in dementia care. *Neurobiology of Aging, 23,* S540.

Smith, S.J. (1998). Providing palliative care for the terminal Alzheimer patient. In L.Volicer & A. Hurley (Eds.), *Hospice care for patients with advanced progressive dementia* (pp. 247–256). New York: Springer Publishing Company.

Taylor, R. (2007). *Alzheimer's from the inside out.* Baltimore: Health Professions Press.

Thomas, W.H. (2004). *The Eden Alternative handbook.* Wimberley, TX: The Eden Alternative.

Volicer, L. (2005). End-of-life care for people with dementia in residential care settings. Alzheimer's Association. Retrieved on line at www.alz.org/research/papers.asp

Volicer, L., McKee, A., & Hewitt, S. (2001). Dementia. *Neurologic Clinics of North America, 19,* 867–885.

Volicer, L., Simard, J., Pupa, J.H., Medrek, R., & Riordan, M.E. (2006). Effect of continuous activity programming on behavioral symptoms of dementia. *Journal of the American Medical Directors Association, 7,* 426–431.

Warden, V., Hurley, A.C., & Volicer, L. (2003). Development and psychometric evaluation of the PAINAD (Pain Assessment in Advanced Dementia) Scale. *Journal of the American Medical Directors Association, 4,* 9–15.

Zweig, S.C. (1997). Cardiopulmonary resuscitation and do-not-resuscitate orders in the nursing home. *Archives of Family Medicine, 6,* 424–429.

Hospice

THE HISTORY OF HOSPICE

The origins of hospice can be traced back to early Western Civilization when the term was used to describe a place of shelter and rest for weary travelers. Notations have been found among the writings of monks caring for warrior knights during the Crusades. They speak of caring for the aged and wounded knights, keeping their bed linens clean, serving warm soup, and washing the feet of the knights. Not much has changed; this comforting care is at the core of current hospice services.

The modern hospice movement began about 1967 at St. Joseph's Hospital in London's East End. It was in this hospital that Dame Cicely Saunders began to experiment with pain medication and symptom relief for terminally ill patients. In 1967, she opened St. Christopher's Hospice, a place of comfort for the terminally ill. This hospice became the model for hospice programs all over the world and mainly served individuals with cancer.

In the United States, Dr. Elisabeth Kübler-Ross began working with terminally ill patients in acute care settings. She found that physicians and other health care workers had difficulty talking about death to these patients. The patients, however, wanted to talk about what was happening to them and wanted to be assured they would be free of pain and would not die alone. In her discussions with dying patients, Kübler-Ross discovered that they usually go through stages in their acceptance of death. She reported her findings in *On Death and Dying*, published in 1969. This book, now considered a classic, heightened public awareness of the loneliness, isolation, and special needs of the dying. As awareness of the special needs of the dying increased, health care professionals and others turned to hospice as a way of caring for people with terminal illnesses.

A group from Yale University visited St. Christopher's Hospice in England and was inspired by what they heard and saw. They resolved to begin a hospice program in the United States. In 1974, a hospice home care program was developed in New Haven, Connecticut. An inpatient center, Connecticut Hospice, Inc., followed in 1980. This was the beginning of the hospice movement in the United States.

There are now thousands of hospice programs in the United States serving millions of people with terminal illnesses and their families. Some have retained their status as voluntary organizations; however, the majority of them are Medicare certified. Most hospice recipients have a diagnosis of cancer with a predictable life expectancy; very few patients have a diagnosis of dementia, primarily because it is difficult to make a prognosis of 6 months of survival, which is required by the Medicare hospice benefit.

Barriers to Identifying Patients with Dementia

Residents in nursing facilities may be the most underserved population among people with terminal illnesses. Although many nursing facility residents die each year in the facility, very few residents with dementia receive services from a Medicare-certified hospice organization. There are many reasons that nursing home residents with advanced dementia continue to be underserved:

- Physicians do not refer their nursing facility patients to hospice because they are uneasy about giving a 6-month survival prognosis. When they realize the resident is actively dying, they believe it is too late to call hospice.

- Many physicians and nursing facility staff feel hospice is a duplication of services already received in the nursing facility.

- Families believe hospice is expensive and do not realize it can be provided in a nursing facility.

- Nursing facilities do not always encourage hospice because it may mean losing Medicare days, which are reimbursed at a higher rate than payments for hospice, which are usually made at the Medicaid rate.

- Nursing facility staff members feel protective of their residents and believe they can provide palliative care themselves.

- Nursing facility staff fears that the survey process might be complicated by having hospice staff involved with residents.

Residents, their families, or their Power of Attorneys (POAs) have the right to be informed about possible eligibility for the Medicare hospice benefit. This topic should be discussed during care plan meetings before the resident actually needs hospice so the family has an opportunity to think about the option before having to make a decision. The facility's social worker should have hospice information available to give families, including those with a loved one in Namaste Care.

MEDICARE HOSPICE BENEFIT

The Medicare hospice benefit was enacted in 1983 to provide palliative care to patients receiving Medicare benefits. At that time, patients had to have a home and a primary caregiver to be eligible, which excluded nursing home residents. In the 1990s, interpretation was changed so that "home" could mean a nursing facility and "caregiver" could mean nursing facility staff. Before a resident in a nursing facility can elect the hospice benefit, the nursing facility must have a contract with a Medicare-approved hospice organization. Most facilities have several contracts so that residents can choose the hospice program with which they want to work.

Medicare Hospice Benefit Criteria

Nursing facility residents must meet the following criteria to be eligible for the Medicare hospice benefit:

- Be eligible for Medicare Part A
- Have 6 months or less to live if the disease follows its expected course, as certified by the attending physician and hospice medical director
- Have a statement, signed by the resident's family or POA, choosing hospice care instead of routine Medicare-covered benefits

for the terminal illness (Medicare continues to pay for health problems not related to the terminal illness)

- Have a contract with a Medicare-approved hospice program

Eligibility for Residents with Alzheimer's Disease

Residents with Alzheimer's disease or a related dementia must meet additional criteria to be eligible for the Medicare hospice benefit:

1. They must be at Stage 7 or beyond, according to the Functional Assessment Staging (FAST) scale, which means they

   - Are unable to ambulate without assistance

   - Cannot dress without assistance

   - Cannot bathe without assistance

   - Experience urinary or fecal incontinence, intermittent or constant

   - Have no meaningful verbal communication, use stereotypical phrases only, or speak six or fewer intelligible words

2. They also must have had one of the following within the past 12 months:

   - Aspiration pneumonia

   - Pyelonephritis or other upper urinary tract infection

   - Septicemia

   - Multiple Stage 3 or 4 decubitus ulcers

   - Fever that recurs after antibiotic therapy

   - Inability to maintain sufficient fluid and calorie intake, with 10% weight loss during the previous 6 months or a serum albumin level less than 2.5 grams per deciliter

HOSPICE SERVICES

Medicare covers the following hospice services and pays almost all of the costs:

- Physician services; residents may continue to use their current attending physician

- Nursing care, including licensed nurses as well as care partners
- Medical equipment
- Medical supplies related to the terminal illness
- Drugs for symptom and pain relief (co-pay is no more than $5 for each prescription if the resident has no other prescription coverage)
- Short-term care in the hospital, including respite and in-patient care for pain and symptom management (resident is responsible for 5% of the Medicare payment for in-patient respite care)
- Home health aide and homemaker services (rarely used for nursing facility residents)
- Physical and occupational therapy (rarely used for patients with advanced dementia)
- Speech therapy (rarely used for patients with advanced dementia)
- Social work services (usually focused on families of patients with advanced dementia)
- Dietary counseling
- Grief and bereavement services for the family for 13 months following the death; this includes individual counseling as well as bereavement support groups
- Volunteer services
- Spiritual care

Hospice does not pay for room and board. If the resident is paying privately, he or she must continue to cover this cost. If Medicaid is the payment source, then it continues to pay the board and room and the payment goes to the hospice, which in turn pays it to the nursing facility. Residents cannot receive Medicare Part A services and hospice in the nursing facility unless the reason for the Part A care is unrelated to the terminal illness.

Medicare Hospice Benefit Periods

When a resident has been accepted for hospice care, he or she is certified for two 90-day periods of care followed by an unlimited number of 60-day periods. This continues as long as the resident remains eligible. Occasionally, a resident will rally; if that happens, the resident would be discharged from hospice and revert to the traditional Medicare program. The resident can return to hospice at any time his or her medical status changes and the resident meets the criteria for hospice. The family or POA always has the option to stop hospice services.

HOSPICE PLAN OF CARE

The nursing facility staff and hospice staff develop an interdisciplinary plan of care for the resident that defines the scope and frequency of hospice services as well as the medical supplies and durable medical equipment that hospice will provide. The hospice plan of care is approved by the facility's attending physician and the hospice medical director; it is reviewed every 2 weeks and updated as necessary. The hospice plan of care is incorporated into the resident's plan of care. Cooperation and communication are the keys to a successful implementation of the joint care plans.

Hospice and Namaste Care

Nursing facilities that offer Namaste Care find that it helps develop stronger ties with the hospice staff and providers. The hospice programs appreciate the emphasis of Namaste Care on a palliative care philosophy for residents with advanced dementia. Namaste Care also makes identifying potential hospice residents easier. A reciprocal arrangement develops when the facility refers residents with advanced dementia to the hospice and the hospice refers families with loved ones who have advanced dementia to the nursing facility.

If the nursing facility has a relationship with hospice organizations, the facility needs to schedule an in-service to explain the Namaste Care program to the hospice staff. Competing hospice programs often vie for the same patients, so the facility might want to meet individually with each hospice program. The educational program should be presented in the facility, giving hospice staff the opportunity to see the program in action if it has been implemented, or to see where it will take place if it is in the planning stage. They can also meet key staff and ask questions about the program. Knowing how Namaste Care works is important for the hospice administrative staff, hospice nurses, and hospice care partners.

The nursing facility staff needs to understand how hospice works as well. It is helpful if one or more hospice organizations provides an in-service on its role in providing care to residents. All facility staff must understand the role of hospice so that when a resident's condition changes, the hospice nurse is called before any action is taken. Hospice would rarely hospitalize one of its patients, for instance. If the nursing facility sends a resident who is receiving hospice benefits to the hospital, a paperwork nightmare ensues for the hospice program. Regular meetings between hospice nurses and facility nurses will help to make the relationship between the two organizations strong.

A special meeting should also be scheduled between the billing departments of the nursing facility and the hospice organization. As soon as a resident elects the hospice benefit, billing changes must be handled in an efficient and timely manner to stay within reimbursement regulations.

The hospice medical director and the facility medical director must share an understanding of each other's regulations. Involving these physicians in the first meetings between hospice and the nursing facility administration is again helpful to strengthen the relationship between the two entities; these physicians should be helping with identifying and approving residents for hospice care. The facility medical director can make sure all attending physicians know the criteria for a hospice referral and that they understand the services that hospice will provide. Some physicians fear a loss of control over their patient if hospice is involved. Physicians may not understand why hospice would be involved with a resident who is in the advanced stage of dementia and, therefore, would not suggest hospice care. It is important to make sure the medical staff understands how helpful hospice staff can be, not only to the resident and the family, but also to the nursing facility staff.

Hospice Services for Namaste Care Residents

When a resident elects the Medicare hospice benefit, hospice staff will provide additional support to the nursing facility staff in several ways:

- Care partners are scheduled to assist with activities of daily living, including feeding and bathing.

- Hospice volunteers are recruited to provide services for the resident, such as taking the person outside in good weather and visiting with him or her in the Namaste Care room. Volunteers may also agree to *sit vigil* for a resident who is actively dying and has no family available, or in instances when the family requests that someone stay with its dying family member.

- Hospice nurses are available for consultation for clinical services.

- Counseling from social workers and clergy is offered to families and staff.

- Medical equipment is available for the resident's comfort, such as special mattresses and lounge chairs.

- 24-hour nursing support is available, especially when needed for pain and discomfort.

- Spiritual services are offered.

Namaste Care provides a unique opportunity for hospice workers providing services to residents with advanced dementia. Hospice care partners should be offered an opportunity to work with the Namaste Care team members. It is important to note that hospice staff is more familiar with patients who are oriented; the staff may therefore appreciate the opportunity to learn about techniques used by Namaste carers to provide meaningful activities for residents with advanced dementia. Hospice and Namaste Care share the same philosophy: a palliative approach to providing care and approaching death with dignity. Working together, this strong partnership benefits residents, their families, and nursing facility staff.

Namaste Care Nursing Supplies

PERSONAL SUPPLIES

Each resident who attends Namaste Care on a regular basis must have a zip-lock plastic bag clearly marked with his or her name. The bag should contain the following personal care items:

- Hairbrush and/or comb
- Nail clipper
- Emory board
- Lip balm
- Any other personal items supplied by the family (e.g., lipstick, additional make-up, hair decorations, after-shave lotion)

GENERAL SUPPLIES

Hair Products

- Combs and/or brushes
- Ribbons, decorative hair combs, other washable hair ornaments for the ladies

Face Products

- Face cream, unscented and nonallergenic (Ponds is a favorite); for infection control, cream must be transferred into individual containers or scooped from the original container using individual Q-tips or other applicators before putting it on residents' faces
- Shaving cream (same infection precautions apply as for face cream)

- Safety razor (must have a safe and appropriate container for disposing of razors)
- Shaving lotion (Old Spice is a favorite); ask the family about the resident's preferred brand of after-shave lotion (the family may provide it)

Mouth Care Products
- Lemon glycerin swab sticks
- Toothette disposable oral swabs
- Lip gloss
- Soft toothbrushes
- Toothpaste

Hand and Fingernail Products
- Basins
- Soap
- Orange sticks
- Emory boards
- Nail clippers

Skin Products
- Baby oil or lotions
- Unscented lotions

Food and Beverages
- Thickeners
- Yogurt
- Ice cream
- Pudding
- Lollipops
- Orange slices

- Crushed pineapple
- Popsicles
- Orange juice
- Cranberry juice
- Soft cookies

Paper Products

- Paper cups
- Covered sip cups
- Flexible straws
- Spoons
- Napkins
- Plastic wrap
- Marker and labels
- Small storage bags
- Paper towels

Linen

- Pillows (for positioning)
- Blankets (colorful)
- Sheets (colorful)
- Quilts
- Face cloths
- Towels

Miscellaneous

- Disposable wipes
- Small plastic bags for individual residents
- Large plastic bags for storing items
- Wastebasket and plastic inserts

- Laundry basket for soiled items
- Latex gloves
- Hand-washing liquid
- Pens and pencils
- Laundry marker
- Notepaper
- Communication book

Namaste Care Activity Supplies

ACTIVITY SUPPLIES

- Stuffed animals, especially soft, realistic birds that make specific bird calls
- Realistic dolls
- Aromatherapy diffuser (must be approved by maintenance department)
- Essential oils, especially lavender
- Scents that reflect different seasons, such as fir and cinnamon for winter, cut grass and flowers for spring/summer, and pumpkin for autumn
- Nature videos
- Sensory materials (e.g., pieces of fabric, silk, satin, leather, rabbit fur, lace, cashmere)
- Antique items (e.g., kitchen implements, marbles, old glass milk bottles, recipe boxes)
- Musical items (e.g., wind chimes, music boxes, rain sticks, drums, bells, singing bowl)
- Q Cord for playing music
- Portable CD/tape player
- Compact disks (CDs) or audiotapes of music and nature sounds
- Tabletop fountains
- Assorted reading material, including spiritual texts, poetry, holiday readings
- Humorous material (e.g., funny hats, circus wigs, realistic animal puppets)
- Sensory balls
- Bubble soap and a bubble machine

Namaste Care Resources

ACTIVITY SUPPLIES

Actron QChord Network
P.O. Box 572244
Tarzana, CA 91357-2244

www.qchord.net
800-866-8887

Nasco
901 Janesville Avenue
P.O. Box 901
Fort Atkinson, WI 53538-0901

www.enasco.com/senioractivities
800-558-9595

S&S Worldwide
75 Mill Street
Colchester, CT 06415

www.ssww.com
800-288-9941

Flaghouse, Inc.
601 FlagHouse Drive
Hasbrouck Heights, NJ 07604-3116

www.flaghouse.com
800-793-7900

Oriental Trading Company
P.O. Box 2308
Omaha, NE 68103-2308

www.orientaltrading.com
800-875-8480

Geriatric Resources, Inc.

www.geriatric-resources.com

Snoezelen

see Flaghouse web site

Mother Earth Pillows
Jenneman Lane
Arnold, MO 63010

www.motherearthpillows.com
800-344-2072

Cedar Lake Productions
445 South Curtis Road
West Allis, WI 53214

www.CedarLakeDVD.com
800-642-8778

Aromatherapy

www.aromaweb.com

NURSING SUPPLIES

Direct Supply   www.DirectSupply.net

ALZHEIMER'S INFORMATION AND EDUCATION

Alzheimer's Association   www.alz.org
(national headquarters)
Information about local Alzheimer's
Association chapters is available on
the national headquarters web site

Alzheimer's Disease Education   www.alzheimers.org
and Referral Center (ADEAR)

SPECIAL RESOURCES

There are numerous web sites devoted to issues surrounding end-of-life care. In addition to the sites listed below, search on any of the following key words with an Internet search engine (e.g., Google):

- Hospice care
- Palliative care
- Death and dying
- Advanced dementia
- End-of-life care

Good Endings   www.goodendings.net

National Hospice and Palliative   www.nhpco.org
Care Organization (NHPCO)

Local hospices are listed in the
yellow pages or on the Internet
(search using the name of your
city followed by *hospice* to find
services in your area).

Namaste Care Checklist

Complete checklist at least once per month.
Write date and initials in top space. Check off each requirement that is met in the column below.

Date and initials								
Namaste Care room								
Soothing music playing								
Lights dimmed								
Chairs for visitors								
Welcome sign on door								
Door clean								
Floor clean								
Chairs clean								
Counters clean								
Kitchen appliances clean								
Furniture clean								
Windows clean								
Window treatments clean and in order								
Wastebasket emptied and tidy								
Quilts and blankets clean and available								
Overall room neat and clutter free								

Plants in good condition							
Other:							
Other:							
Namaste Care residents							
Look comfortable and peaceful, no groaning or anxious facial expressions							
Faces clean and moistened							
Hair groomed							
No unpleasant odor in the room or with any particular resident							
Hands clean							
Fingernails clean							
Arms moisturized							
Legs moisturized							
Clothing clean							
Blanket or quilt clean							
Other:							
Other:							
Namaste Care supplies							
Hand cream							
Face cream							
Shaving cream							
After-shave lotion							
Safety razors							
Mouth care items							
Combs/brushes							
Lavender and essential oils							

Seasonal scents							
Stuffed birds and other animals available							
Lollipops available							
Orange slices and other foods available							
Plastic bags, small and large							
Other:							
Other:							
Namaste Care infection control							
Refrigerator clean and set to correct temperature							
Refrigerator temperature log current							
Food dated							
Beverages available							
Gloves used by staff handling food							
Hand-washing supplies							
Separate containers for resident personal supplies							
Individual blanket/quilt per resident							
Soiled laundry in closed container							
Electric items inspected by Maintenance							
Other:							
Other:							
Namaste Care team member							
Name tag visible							
Greets everyone entering room							
Monitors resident safety							

Interacts with residents							
Always present in room							
Other:							
Other:							

The Namaste Care Team Staff Interview

[Begin the interview with a brief overview of the program and expectations.]

Thank you for your interest in becoming part of the Namaste Care team!

The success of any program depends on the commitment of the people who work on it. In assembling the Namaste Care team, we realize that working with residents who have advanced dementia is not for everyone. We are looking for individuals who want to join the Namaste Care team and who have the desire to be part of an exciting new concept in dementia care.

The purpose of this interview is not to judge your job performance; it is an opportunity for you to understand the expectations of being a Namaste Care team member so that you can make an informed decision about whether to be a part of this program. We also want to make sure you understand the philosophy of Namaste Care and your role in helping to provide a quality of life for residents with advanced dementia. Namaste Care is based on a social model of care as opposed to a medical model.

[Provide staff with a copy of the Namaste Care philosophy statement and/or mission statement.]

The [name of facility or dementia program] believes the following:

- Excellent nursing care should be provided to all residents.
- The dignity of every resident must be honored and be a priority for all staff.
- Residents are pain free and comfortable around the clock.
- Comfort care is practiced.

- Families are supported.
- Because residents can no longer self-initiate activities, the staff must help them continue to be engaged with meaningful activities throughout their waking hours. It is the responsibility of all staff to be involved in activities. ADLs are not approached as tasks but as opportunities for meaningful interaction.

Namaste Care will grow and develop in ways we cannot imagine, therefore Namaste Care team members are

- Flexible and willing to try new approaches
- Able to give and receive constructive feedback
- Capable of bringing joy to their work

NAMASTE CARE QUESTIONNAIRE

The following questions have been developed to help you determine if being a part of the Namaste Care team is for you. Please take a few moments to respond to each question.

1. What do you think is the difference between a social model and a medical model of care? _____

   _____

   _____

   _____

2. How long have you worked in a nursing facility? _____

3. How long have you worked at [name of facility]? _____

4. What do you like about your work? _____

   _____

5. What is your experience of working with people with dementia?

   _____

   _____

   _____

6. What attracts you to the Namaste Care team?

   _____

   _____

_____

_____

_____

7. What do you believe makes a team work well together?

_____

_____

_____

8. Describe one of the most enjoyable times you have experienced with a resident. _____

_____

_____

9. How do you approach a resident who does not want to do something, such as take a bath or get dressed?

_____

_____

_____

10. What are your feelings about working with residents in the last stage of dementia who will die while in your care?

_____

_____

_____

_____

11. Describe a "good death."

_____

_____

_____

12. When your assigned duties are complete, what do you do if you have some free time?

_____

_____

_____

Expectations for being a part of the Namaste Care team include:

- Maintaining excellent attendance and understanding that the Namaste Care team and residents are affected when assigned staff members do not come to work
- Assisting in the Namaste Care room as time allows
- Assisting with hydration and feeding
- Filling in for the Namaste Care specialist
- Being open to trying new approaches and activities
- Having fun and knowing that you make a difference in the lives of residents in Namaste Care

Your comments:

_____

_____

_____

_____

_____

_____

_____

_____

_____

_____

_____

_____

"I understand Namaste Care and the expectations of team members. I would like to be a member of the Namaste Care team."

_____   _____
Signature   Date

Gifts of Love Letter and Flyer

GIFTS OF LOVE LETTER (SAMPLE)

Dear Friends,

The Vermont Veterans Home has been caring for those who have served our country for more than 100 years. Our dementia program has been recognized for its innovation and excellence throughout this country and was featured at the International Alzheimer's Conference in Sweden.

It is somewhat ironic that we have chosen to begin a program focusing on the residents with advanced Alzheimer's disease or a related dementia at a time when much-loved former president Ronald Reagan began his last journey with Alzheimer's disease. President Reagan and his family have experienced the despair and sadness that touches everyone who loves a person with Alzheimer's disease.

More than 4 million Americans have Alzheimer's disease. This disease touches the rich and the poor, men and women. It does not respect status, race, or religion. Although closer to finding the cause or causes and possible cures, we cannot stop this disease. Thousands die from complications of Alzheimer's disease each year.

The Vermont Veterans Home has developed a unique program called Namaste Care. This program promises to help our residents and their families face the last stage of the disease within a supportive, family-like setting that focuses on comfort care and a quality of life until the end of life.

(continued)

(continued)

We need the help of the Bennington community to make this final home look and feel like a home. We ask you to read the attached description of Namaste Care and the "Gifts of Love" project and then ask yourself how you can offer your veterans a gift of love.

On behalf of the staff and residents of The Vermont Veterans Home, thank you.

Administrator's Name

GIFTS OF LOVE FLYER (SAMPLE)

NAMASTE CARE

The Namaste Care program is a program for residents of The Vermont Veterans Home who are in the advanced stage of Alzheimer's disease or a related progressive dementia. This unique program offers a comfort care approach to end-of-life care and is one component of The Vermont Veterans Home's dementia program.

The Namaste Care program is named after an Eastern Indian term that means "to honor the spirit within." It is the final home for many veterans. The Vermont Veterans Home has dedicated a 17-bed unit on C Wing for the purpose of creating a quiet, calming environment for residents and their families to find peace in this last stage of their journey into Alzheimer's disease.

As a nonprofit facility dedicated to providing quality care for military veterans in Vermont, we are counting on the Bennington community for help in making the Namaste Care unit as comfortable and home-like as possible.

The Gifts of Love project needs the people of Bennington, especially the many artists and businesses, to donate gifts of love. These gifts may include artwork and items such as handmade quilts that reflect the peace and tranquility of our program.

We are also in need of furniture and carpeting for a family room where families of our residents who are in the last days of life can relax and rest.

(continued)

(continued)

Directly across from the family room we have dedicated one room, the Reagan Room, as a place where residents in their final days of life may stay in a quiet, private place with their families. To transform this room into a home-like bedroom, we need donations to purchase bedroom furniture and a sleeping couch or chair for family members wishing to stay overnight and be close to their loved one. Contributions of carpeting, special linens, pictures, and draperies will all help to make a difficult experience easier for families and the residents.

If you feel you could give a "gift of love" to the veterans who have served our country so valiantly in the past, please call [Name of director] at [phone number].

Alzheimer's Disease Bill of Rights

The Alzheimer's Disease Bill of Rights

Every person diagnosed with Alzheimer's disease
or a related disorder deserves the following rights:

To be informed of one's diagnosis

To have appropriate, ongoing medical care

To be productive in work and play for as long as possible

To be treated like an adult, not like a child

To have expressed feelings taken seriously

To be free from psychotropic medications, if possible

To live in a safe, structured, and predictable environment

To enjoy meaningful activities that fill each day

To be outdoors on a regular basis

To have physical contact, including
hugging, caressing, and hand-holding

To be with individuals who know one's life story,
including cultural and religious traditions

To be cared for by individuals
who are well trained in dementia care

Source: Bell, V., & Troxel, D. (2003). The Best Friends approach to Alzheimer's care. *Baltimore: Health Professions Press. Reprinted with permission.*

APPENDIX I

Pain Assessment in Advanced Dementia (PAINAD) Scale

	0	1	2	Score
Breathing (independent of vocalization)	Normal	Occasional labored breathing Short period of hyperventilation	Noisy labored breathing Long period of hyperventilation Cheyne-Stokes respiration	
Negative Vocalization	None	Occasional moan or groan Low level speech with a negative or disapproving quality	Repeated, troubled calling out Loud moaning or groaning Crying	
Facial Expression	Smiling, or inexpressive	Sad Frightened Frowning	Facial grimacing	
Body Language	Relaxed	Tense Distressed pacing Fidgeting	Rigid Clenched fists Knees pulled up Pulling or pushing away Striking out	
Consolability	No need to console	Distracted or reassured by voice or touch	Unable to console, distract, or reassure	
				TOTAL

Signature _____

Source: Warden, V., Hurley, A.C., & Volicer, L. (2003). Development and psychometric evaluation of the PAINAD (Pain Assessment in Advanced Dementia) Scale. Journal of the American Medical Directors Association, 4, 9–15. *Reprinted with permission.*

KEY

Breathing

1. *Normal breathing* is characterized by effortless, quiet, rhythmic (smooth) respirations.

2. *Occasional labored breathing* is characterized by episodic bursts of harsh, difficult, or straining respirations.

3. *Short period of hyperventilation* is characterized by intervals of rapid, deep breaths lasting a short period of time.

4. *Noisy labored breathing* is characterized by negative sounding respirations on inhalation or exhalation. These may be loud, gurgling, or wheezing and appear strenuous or straining.

5. *Long period of hyperventilation* is characterized by an excessive rate and depth of respiration lasting a considerable time.

6. *Cheyne-Stokes respiration* is characterized by rhythmic waxing and waning of breathing, from very deep to shallow respirations with periods of apnea (cessation of breathing).

Negative Vocalization

1. *None* is characterized by speech or vocalization that has a neutral or pleasant quality.

2. *Occasional moan or groan* is characterized by mournful or murmuring sounds, wails, or laments. Groaning is characterized by louder than usual, inarticulate involuntary sounds, often abruptly beginning and ending.

3. *Low level speech with a negative or disapproving quality* is characterized by muttering, mumbling, whining, grumbling, or swearing in a low volume with a complaining, sarcastic, or caustic tone.

4. *Repeated, troubled calling out* is characterized by phrases or words being used over and over in a tone that suggests anxiety, uneasiness, or distress.

5. *Loud moaning or groaning* is characterized by mournful or murmuring sounds, wails, or laments in much louder than usual

volume. Loud groaning is characterized by louder than usual inarticulate, involuntary sounds, often abruptly beginning and ending.

6. *Crying* is characterized by an utterance of emotion accompanied by tears. There may be sobbing or quiet weeping.

Facial Expression

1. *Smiling or inexpressive* is characterized by either upturned corners of the mouth, brightening of the eyes, and a look of pleasure or contentment or a neutral, at-ease, relaxed, or blank look.

2. *Sad* is characterized by an unhappy, lonesome, sorrowful, or dejected look. There may be tears in the eyes.

3. *Frightened* is characterized by a look of fear, alarm, or heightened anxiety. Eyes appear wide open.

4. *Frown* is characterized by a downward turn of the corners of the mouth. Increased facial wrinkling in the forehead and around the mouth may appear.

5. *Facial grimacing* is characterized by a distorted, distressed look. The brow is more wrinkled, as is the area around the mouth. Eyes may be squeezed shut.

Body Language

1. *Relaxed* is characterized by a calm, restful, mellow appearance. The person seems to be taking it easy.

2. *Tense* is characterized by a strained, apprehensive, or worried appearance. The jaw may be clenched (exclude any contractures).

3. *Distressed pacing* is characterized by activity that seems unsettled. There may be a fearful, worried, or disturbed element present. The rate of walking may by faster or slower.

4. *Fidgeting* is characterized by restless movement. Squirming about or wiggling in the chair or bed may occur. The person might be hitching a chair across the room. Repetitive touching, tugging, or rubbing of body parts can also be observed.

5. *Rigid* is characterized by stiffening of the body. The arms and/or legs are tight and inflexible. The trunk may appear straight and unyielding (exclude any contractures).

6. *Clenched fists* is characterized by tightly closed hands. They may be opened and closed repeatedly or held tightly shut.

7. *Knees pulled up* is characterized by flexing the legs and drawing the knees up toward the chest. May occur with an overall troubled appearance (exclude any contractures).

8. *Pulling or pushing away* is characterized by resistiveness upon approach or to care. The person is trying to escape by yanking or wrenching him- or herself free or by shoving the caregiver away.

9. *Striking out* is characterized by hitting, kicking, grabbing, punching, biting, or other forms of personal assault.

Consolability

1. *No need to console* is characterized by a sense of well-being. The person appears content.

2. *Distracted or reassured by voice or touch* is characterized by a disruption in the distressed behavior when the person is spoken to or touched. The behavior stops during the period of interaction, with no further indication that the person is distressed.

3. *Unable to console, distract, or reassure* is characterized by the inability to sooth the person or stop a behavior with words or actions. No amount of comforting—verbal or physical—will alleviate the behavior.

Index